MAMMOGRAPHY EXAM REVIEW

MAMMOGRAPHY EXAM REVIEW

Jennifer R. Wagner

Erica Koch Wight

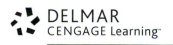
DELMAR
CENGAGE Learning™

Australia Canada Mexico Singapore Spain United Kingdom United States

Mammography Exam Review
by
Jennifer R. Wagner, R.T.(R)(M)(QM)
Erica Koch Wight, M.Ed.,
R.T.(R)(M)(QM)

Vice President, Health Care
  Business Unit: **William Brottmiller**

Director of Learning Solutions:
  Matthew Kane

Acquisitions Editor: **Kalen Conerly**

Product Manager: **Natalie Pashoukos**

Editorial Assistant: **Meaghan O'Brien**

Marketing Director: **Jennifer McAvey**

Marketing Manager: **Michele McTighe**

Marketing Coordinator:
  Chelsey Iaquinta

Technology Director: **Mary Colleen
  Liburdi**

Production Director: **Carolyn Miller**

Senior Art Director: **Jack Pendleton**

Content Project Manager: **Katie Wachtl**

Technology Project Manager:
  Patti Allen

For product information and technology assistance, contact us at
Professional & Career Group Customer Support, 1-800-648-7450

For permission to use material from this text or product, submit all requests online at **www.cengage.com/permissions**
Further permissions questions can be emailed to
permissionrequest@cengage.com

Library of Congress Control Number
2007039755

ISBN 10: 1-4180-5079-2
ISBN 13: 978-1-4180-5079-5

Delmar Cengage Learning
5 Maxwell Drive
Clifton Park, NY 12065-2919
USA

Cengage Learning products are represented in Canada by Nelson Education, Ltd.

For your lifelong learning solutions, visit **delmar.cengage.com**

Visit our corporate website at **www.cengage.com**

Notice to the Reader
Publisher does not warrant or guarantee any of the products described herein or perform any independent analysis in connection with any of the product information contained herein. Publisher does not assume, and expressly disclaims, any obligation to obtain and include information other than that provided to it by the manufacturer. The reader is expressly warned to consider and adopt all safety precautions that might be indicated by the activities described herein and to avoid all potential hazards. By following the instructions contained herein, the reader willingly assumes all risks in connection with such instructions. The publisher makes no representations or warranties of any kind, including but not limited to, the warranties of fitness for particular purpose or merchantability, nor are any such representations implied with respect to the material set forth herein, and the publisher takes no responsibility with respect to such material. The publisher shall not be liable for any special, consequential, or exemplary damages resulting, in whole or part, from the readers' use of, or reliance upon, this material.

Printed in the United States of America
1 2 3 4 5 6 7 8 11 10 09 08 07

Contents

1

Patient Education and Assessment   1

Instrumentation and Quality Assurance   15

Anatomy, Physiology, and Pathology   37

Mammographic Techniques and Image Evaluation   53

Breast Positioning and Special Procedures   61

Practice Examination   75

Internet Resources and Bibliography   93

Index   95

Preface

The importance of quality mammography in the field of medical imaging cannot be underestimated. This textbook was developed to meet a need in the industry to see more registry review content for those wishing to take the American Registry of Radiologic Technologists (ARRT) advanced examination in Mammography. It is designed to serve as a guide and a reference for the registered radiologic technologist wishing to become a qualified mammographer.

The text is constructed to model the newest ARRT content specifications for Mammography. Subject matter includes digital imaging, methods of breast biopsy, quality control, breast positioning and technique, pathology, patient care, and instrumentation. The text covers key points of the five content areas of the exam: Patient Education and Assessment; Instrumentation and Quality Assurance; Anatomy, Physiology, and Pathology; Mammographic Technique and Image Evaluation; and Positioning and Interventional Procedures. However, it is the hope of the authors that the reader will use as much reference material as possible when studying for the examination, not this text solely.

ORGANIZATION OF THE TEXT

As stated previously, the text models the content specifications for the Mammography examination administered by the ARRT. Chapters 1 through 5 cover Patient Education and Assessment; Instrumentation and Quality Assurance; Anatomy, Physiology, and Pathology; Mammographic Technique and Image Evaluation; and Positioning and Interventional Procedures. Each chapter begins with an overview on the specific content area and ends with practice questions formatted in the style of the registry exam. Answers with detailed explanations are also included at the end of each chapter.

Chapter 6 is a written practice examination weighted similarly to the ARRT exam to help readers identify areas that need additional study.

Line drawings and radiographs are included throughout the text to help readers visualize positioning techniques, pathology of the breast, and diagnostic comparisons.

SUPPLEMENTS

Also included with the text is a free CD-ROM with over 300 additional questions to assist in review of the various content areas. The CD is organized in two parts: a study mode and a practice test mode. The program randomly selects questions from this large available pool, and each time you start a new study session or a new practice test, you get a new assortment of questions.

The text was designed to enhance skills in taking tests by using a multiple choice question format as well as multiple choice questions with images in order to assist the reader in exam preparation. Since the ARRT examination is computerized, the digital media are included to allow the reader the experience of the computerized examination environment.

It is the authors' hope that this resource will enhance the quality of exam review and help better prepare mammographers for the field.

About the Authors

Jennifer Wagner is a faculty member in the Medical Diagnostic Imaging Program at Fort Hays State University in Hays, Kansas. Her teaching experience spans across Radiology, Mammography, and Ultrasound.

Erica Koch Wight is the Program Director for the Medical Imaging Program at the University of Alaska Anchorage. She has many years of experience in Imaging and Mammography.

Acknowledgments

We wish to acknowledge Margaret Gallo, R.T.(R)(M)(QM), QC/QA Technologist, Woman's Hospital, Baton Rouge, Louisiana for generously providing a good majority of the images for this text. We are especially grateful for the assistance of our editor, Kalen Conerly, for her encouragement and assistance in preparing the manuscript. We could not have put together this text without the support of Natalie Pashoukos, our Product Manager at Delmar.

We appreciate the constant support of our families and colleagues with this project, as many weekends and nights were dedicated to making the project a success.

Reviewers

Jan Gillespie Clark, M.Ed., R.T. (R)(CV)(M)(QM)
Trainer III
WellPoint-Health Management Corporation
Richmond, Virginia

Catherine Cooper, MS, R.T. (R, CT)
Instructor
University of South Alabama
Mobile, Alabama

Margaret Gallo, R.T. (R)(M)(QM)
Quality Control Technologist
Woman's Hospital Breast Cancer
Baton Rouge, Louisiana

Ellyn Hodgis, M.Ed., R.T., (R)(M)
Assistant Professor - Radiologic Technology
Tidewater Community College
Virginia Beach, Virginia

Linda Pearson, PhD, ARRT, (R)(M)(QM)
Radiologic Technology Program Director
Carl Albert State College
Poteau, Oklahoma

Paulette Peterson, R.T. (R)(M)(QM), M.Ed.
Associate Professor
Monroe Community College
Rochester, New York

Judy Speer, BS, R.T. (R)(M)
Mammography Coordinator/Instructor
Greenville Technical College
Greenville, South Carolina

Christa Weigel, MSRS, ET (R)(M)(BD)
Instructor
Fort Hays State University
Hays, Kansas

Patient Education and Assessment

SIGNIFICANT ASPECTS OF BREAST DISEASE

Risk

Breast cancer risk is associated with a few key, or major factors. First and foremost is gender. Women are more likely to acquire breast cancer; according to the latest statistics from the American Cancer Society, the average lifetime risk is that one in eight women will develop cancer in her lifetime.

The second risk factor is age. The American Cancer Society states that about 17% of invasive breast cancer diagnosed are among women in their 40s, while about 78% of women with invasive breast cancer are age 50 or older when they are diagnosed. Genetic risk accounts for approximately 5–10% of all breast cancers. Having a mother, sister, or daughter with breast cancer doubles one's risk. Having cancer in one breast increases the risk of developing cancer in the other breast by three to four times. Women who had early onset of menses and late onset of menopause have been linked to having a slightly increased risk of breast cancer. This is also true for women who do not have children or have children after age 30. It is found that during the monthly cycle, a woman's fluctuating hormone levels cause changes within breast tissue. These changes possibly encourage or amplify abnormalities in the cell repair processes within breast tissue.

Other conditions that may increase breast cancer risk are the presence of different types of cancer. The American Cancer Society suggests that women who have relatives with breast and ovarian cancer may have a higher incidence of breast and ovarian cancers.

Women may also see an increased risk if they have had previous biopsies which have proven noncancerous conditions. The hyperplasia associated with these conditions has been associated with the development of breast cancer at a later date.

Studies have shown that moderate alcohol consumption may increase breast cancer risk up to 30%. While risk associated with obesity and diet has not been well documented, there are concerns it is linked to breast cancer. It is known that countries with lower fat diets have less incidence of breast cancer. There is a link between estradoil and body fat. It is found that by lowering fat intake, estradoil may be lowered. Estradoil is a form of blood estrogen that has been linked to a higher risk of breast cancer.

Early Detection

Breast cancer is the most commonly diagnosed cancer among American women, except for skin cancer. It is second only to lung cancer as the most common cause of death among women. Mammography is the best available method to detect breast cancer in its earliest, most treatable stage. According to the American Cancer Society and the American College of Radiography, women aged 40 years or older should have a screening mammogram every year. All women should have a baseline mammogram between the ages of 30 and 40 years.

A mammogram will recognize changes in the breast at its early stages thus adding more information about the breast to aid in diagnosis. Early detection is applying a strategy that makes it possible to diagnose breast cancer earlier. Breast cancers that are detected because they are felt by the patient are usually larger and are more likely to have spread. Breast cancer found through early screening is usually small and tends to not have moved beyond the breast.

BSE

Breast self-examination, BSE, is a technique highly encouraged in order for a patient to understand the location and feel of the breast tissue and to recognize changes in her own breast. BSE should be done standing, either in or out of the shower, or lying supine on a bed. Patients with larger breasts usually complete BSE while lying supine. Examining the breast in the upright position allows for better palpation of the superior half of the breast while the supine position will allow for better palpation of the inferior half of the breast. Patients with larger breasts may have better palpation lying supine. The methods suggested by the American Cancer Society are the wedge, circular, and up-and-down. The best time to perform the BSE is immediately after the menstrual period when the breasts are least tender. Those with no regular cycles should perform BSE the same day of each month as per the American Cancer Society.

There are a few easy steps utilized (Figure 1–1):

1. The patient will want to look at the breasts in the mirror and observe their symmetry and position. This should be done each month to note any changes.

2. The patient should be instructed to lie on her back on a bed, and elevate the ipsilateral arm of the breast being examined, for instance the right. Take the pads of the first three fingers of the left hand, not the thumb, and gently, but with some pressure, use one of the suggested methods and move around the right breast. The same method should be used on the left breast.

Repeat the examination on both breasts while standing. Using soapy water sometimes makes the tactile feeling more sensitive, and the examination more effective.

BSE should be part of breast health and recommended to be completed on a monthly basis. Patients younger than 40 years should have a clinical breast examination (CBE) every 3 years. Women over the age of 40 should have a CBE and mammogram every year as per the American Cancer Society Guidelines.

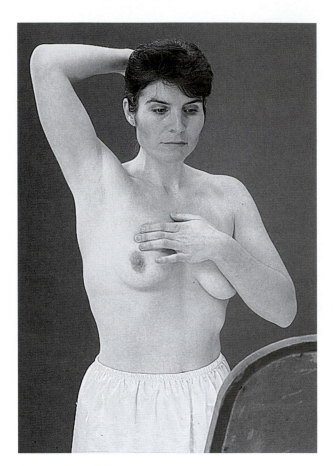

Figure 1–1   BSE

PATIENT HISTORY

The patient history form (Figure 1–2) is one of the most important aspects in the mammography screening process. It is documentation that will aid the radiologist in interpretation of the images. The patient history form should include a diagram of the breasts which can be used to mark any scars, lumps, moles, or other skin aberrations. The history form should also include information on patient history of familial cancer, hormone therapy, and prior breast surgeries to include biopsy. Valuable information includes years of menarche and number of pregnancies.

HORMONAL CHANGES

Hormonal changes in a patient produce some minor risk factors. As discussed before, patients who have started menarche early may have a higher predisposition to breast cancer. Also women who have not

Breast History Form ABC Clinic

Name: _____   Date: _____

Date of Birth: _____   Age: _____

Address: _____

_____

Day Phone: _____   Evening Phone: _____

Could you be pregnant? ❑ Yes   ❑ No *Inform the technologist if you are or think you are pregnant.*

How do you prefer to be contacted, if it should be necessary? _____

Have you had a breast exam by a doctor, nurse, or PA within the past 12 months? ❑ Yes   ❑ No

Have you had a mammogram before? ❑ Yes   ❑ No When? _____   Where? _____

Please circle ROUTINE or RIGHT (R) or LEFT (L)   BREAST HISTORY- Have your ever had

Reason for today's mammogram:

ROUTINE		( ) breast cancer R L date _____
I feel a lump.	R L	( ) breast biopsy R L date _____
I feel a thickening	R L	result _____
My doctor feels something	R L	( ) cyst aspiration R L date _____
Nipple discharge	R L	( ) cyst removed R L date _____
New nipple change	R L	( ) breast reduction R L date _____
Pain	R L	( ) abscess treated R L date _____
Follow something on prior	R L	( ) breast implant R L date _____

Last menstrual period _____ If you have stopped having periods, at what age did they stop? _____

Have you had your ovaries removed? ❑ Yes   ❑ No   Year: _____

Have you had ovarian carcinoma? ❑ Yes   ❑ No

HORMONE USE

Have you ever used female hormones (including vaginal creams, suppositories, or patches) such as estrogen
❑ Yes   ❑ No

If you have, between what ages? _____ to _____ Are you presently using them?
❑ Yes   ❑ No

FAMILY HISTORY (Please circle and *indicate* age at which breast cancer was diagnosed)

Who has had breast cancer? No one Mother ____ Sister ____ Maternal aunt/grandmother ____ Daughter ____

Who has had ovarian carcinoma? No one Mother ____ Sister ____ Maternal aunt/grandmother ____ Daughter ____

BREAST CANCER TREATMENT (Please circle)

Have you had a mastectomy or lumpectomy? ❑ Yes   ❑ No If yes, which side? RIGHT   LEFT

Have you ever had radiation therapy to your breasts? ❑ Yes   ❑ No If yes, when? _____

Have you ever had chemotherapy for breast cancer? ❑ Yes   ❑ No If yes, when? _____

TECHNOLOGIST COMMENTS: TECHNOLOGIST USE ONLY: SCARS AND SKIN LESIONS

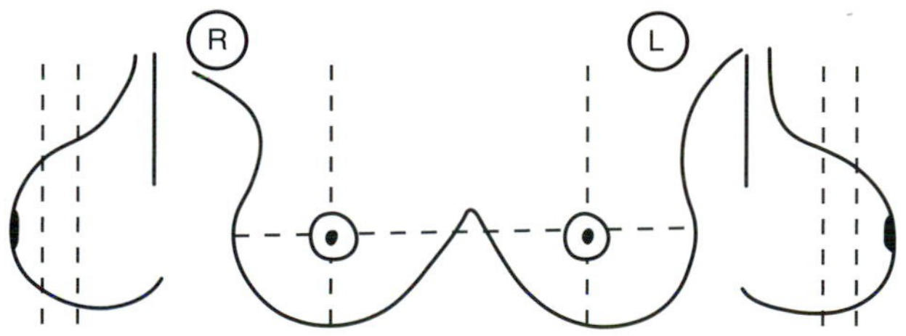

_____

_____

_____

_____

Figure 1–2   Mammography Screening Process

had children or who undergo late menopause may be at higher risk. This is mainly due to hormones and their effect on the breast tissue. Because hormones increase the density of breast tissue, hormone replacement therapy and birth control pills are also thought to have a slight effect on the density of the breast.

BENIGN BREAST DISEASE

These will be discussed in detail under "Anatomy, Physiology, and Pathology."

Benign diseases are those that are noncancerous. Benign tumors do not grow and spread the way malignant tumors do. They are usually not as great a threat. Rarely, these conditions can cause bothersome symptoms. Types of benign breast disease include cysts, lipomas, fibroadenomas, abscesses, gynecomastia, fibrocystic changes, radial scar, and ductal ectasia.

MALIGNANT BREAST DISEASE

Breast cancer is predominantly found in women. A very small percentage, about 1200 new cases each year, of men will develop breast cancer. Breast cancer will arise mainly from glandular tissue. Glandular tissue is usually found toward the central lateral portion of the breast (Figure 1–3). Carcinoma in situ is the most common carcinoma found in the breast. It is usually found in the early stages of its development and is termed in situ because it has not left the duct or lobe. Lobular carcinoma occurs in the lobules of the breast; ductal carcinoma occurs in the ducts of the breast.

SIGNS AND SYMPTOMS OF DISEASE

Identifying abnormalities of the breast is critical for prognosis and treatment options. There are many physical changes in the breast that may point to breast disease. The following are just a few of the more common:

- **Erythema** or redness of the skin usually signifies an inflammatory process, sometimes an inflammatory cancer.
- **Inversion of the nipples**, if not developmentally related, can sometimes signify a tumor.
- **Edema** is a development of fluid within the skin. It creates an orange peel effect of "peau d'orange" and usually indicates an inflammatory carcinoma.
- **Discharge** may be caused by fibrocystic conditions or hormonal fluctuations. Usually the color of the discharge is important, as a clear discharge may signify a cancer.
- **Symmetry**, both breasts should be relatively similar, without pain or unilateral lumps.
- **Pain** is not normally associated with breast cancer. Most women will experience some sort of benign breast pain.

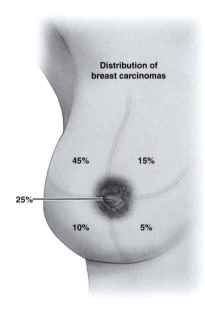

Figure 1–3   Breast Cancer Occurence by Quadrant

- **Dimpling** of the skin is associated with breast cancer. This is a physical sign of underlying pathology.

DIAGNOSTIC OPTIONS

Ultrasonography

The two most prevalent diagnostic tools are mammography and ultrasonography.

Sonography is a secondary option and should not be substituted for mammography. Breast ultrasound is used to determine whether a lump is a cyst (containing fluid) or a solid mass. Fluid is typically withdrawn from a cyst using a needle and syringe. If clear fluid is removed and the mass completely disappears, no further treatment or evaluation is needed.

Sonography can also be used to locate the position of a known tumor in order to guide the physician during a biopsy or aspiration procedure. Sonography, used as a secondary screening tool alongside mammography can bring the number of cancers detected up, especially in women who have dense breasts. Many doctors are now suggesting that screening breast ultrasound be used in conjunction with the mammogram for greater diagnostic abilities.

Biopsy

Biopsy is also an option with some pathologies. A biopsy is the removal of cells or tissues so they can be viewed under a microscope by a pathologist to check for signs of cancer. If a lump in the breast is found, the doctor may need to cut out a small piece of the lump. There are three basic biopsy procedures: fine needle aspiration (FNA), core biopsy, and needle localization.

Needle localizations are usually performed on nonpalpable lesions that will be surgically evaluated. The needle localization allows identification of the area to be excised. The needle localization is performed using mammography. The radiologist and mammographer localize the lesion. The surgeon then takes the patient to the operating room and removes the lesion. Once excised, the sample (specimen) is sent back to the mammography department to be radiographed. This radiograph is used to help ensure the entire pathology has been removed.

FNA requires the use of a very small needle. It is used to aspirate small lesions identified on the mammogram and/or ultrasound. The procedure may be performed under ultrasound guidance, mammographic guidance, or clinical guidance. The FNA technique is used for both palpable and nonpalpable lesions. Cellular material is withdrawn through a needle and then undergoes a pathologic evaluation by the pathologist.

Core biopsy involves removing breast tissue. Core biopsy may be done using different methods. While more current systems are tables, there are still many upright mammography units and attachments used. Core biopsy may be performed with a dedicated stereotactic unit or a hand-held biopsy gun with ultrasound guidance. The stereotactic method is very commonly used for nonpalpable mammographic abnormalities. The patient is positioned lying prone on the stereotactic table. The table uses precise coordinates to locate the area of interest. Once the lesion is triangulated, a tissue sample is obtained by firing a computer-guided 14-gauge needle. A successful fire will produce a 20 mm cylindrical sample of tissue 2 mm in diameter. Several passes may be made, each acquiring a new core sample of tissue. Sometimes a small metallic marker or clip is left in the breast at the biopsy site if further surgical procedure is required. Specimen imaging is still utilized to evaluate the tissue samples removed to identify the presence of microcalcifications. The stereotactic procedure is minimally invasive for the patient. This is a main advantage of this procedure. It will not require a hospital stay, nor will it in most cases produce scarring or require stitches. Some patients may develop a hematoma from the biopsy. There are also risks of infection. Patients should be made well aware of these risks before the procedure.

Ultrasound guided core biopsy utilizes a small hollow-cored needle or vacuum assisted biopsy device. The area of interest is localized with ultrasound. The most common way is to use the vacuum assisted technology. There are two companies that currently make the technology, and the procedures are usually referred to by their brand name, either the Mammotome™ or the MIBB (Minimally Invasive Breast Biopsy).

Ductography

Ductography (also called galactography or ductogalactography) is used to identify anomalies of the duct specifically in patients with nipple discharge. Papillomas are the most common cause of nipple discharge. Other lesions such as ductal carcinoma in situ (DCIS) can also be identified. Before the procedure, the nipple is cleaned and prepared using sterile technique. The radiologist applies pressure to the breast to identify the duct that is producing the discharge. The duct is then cannulated. Methylene blue dye is used when surgical excision is necessary. It is injected into the duct to aid in visualization. A mammogram is taken and any anomalies in the isolated duct are then visualized. The anomaly will appear dark on the mammogram while the contrast-filled duct appears white.

Pneumocystography

Pneumocystography uses aspiration to reduce a cystic lesion in the breast under ultrasound guidance. Fluid is withdrawn from the cyst and an equal amount of air is reinjected to the cyst to allow for wall interrogation. The patient is then imaged with mammography.

MRI

MRI is a modality used as a secondary tool to visualize anomalies in the breast already identified with mammography. It is also used to image patients with breast implants when mammography is not a feasible option. The patient is placed in a strong magnetic field. MRI has high sensitivity for lesions smaller than 1 cm but low specificity of lesions. The limitations of MRI include cost and potential patient physical and emotional inabilities, for instance, claustrophobia.

Sentinel Node Mapping

Sentinel node mapping is also termed lymphoscintigraphy. It is predominantly used to determine whether cancer has spread to the lymph nodes. This is a technique in which a small amount of a radioactive substance is injected into the area surrounding the tumor. The substance will highlight the tumor and will travel toward the area of interest. Because the sentinel lymph node is the first lymph node that filters the fluid draining away from the primary tumor, it is assumed that if this first node contains cancer cells the other lymph nodes may be positive for cancer spread. This sentinel node will help predict the possibility of cancer spread into the remaining surrounding nodes.

TREATMENT OPTIONS

Breast cancer should be treated by a team of health care professionals with experience in treating patients with breast cancer. Breast cancer has a variety of treatment options. Some of the most common factors affecting the options are

- What is the type of cancer?
- What is the stage of the cancer? Has it spread?
- Is it positive for estrogen cancer reception?

- Is this recurrent or recently diagnosed?
- What are the age, health, and menopausal status of the patient?

There are four standard treatment options used. They include surgery, radiation therapy, chemotherapy, and hormone therapy. These are known as adjuvant therapy. Adjuvant therapies are targeted therapies or a combination of therapies that are used to destroy any cancer cells.

Most patients with breast cancer will have surgery to remove a portion or all of the breast tissue. The extent of the tumor will determine the surgical options. There are conservative breast surgeries that include lumpectomy, partial mastectomy, and segmental mastectomy. A total mastectomy will remove all the breast tissue and may remove some of the lymph nodes under the arm. Another type of mastectomy is the radical mastectomy, which removes a portion of the lining over the chest muscles and part of the chest wall muscles.

Lymph node dissection may be done with any breast surgery. It involves removal of the lymph nodes under the arm for dissection.

Treatment of cancer is dependent on some basic things. They include

1. size of tumor
2. stage of tumor
3. tumor location
4. hormone receptor tests

Chemotherapy

Chemotherapy, hormonal therapy, or radiation therapy are used to kill any cancer cells that may be left after surgery. Chemotherapy involves cytotoxic administration of drugs to specifically kill the cancer cells. The type, length, and intensity of the chemotherapy treatment will be dependent upon the cancer type and its stage.

Hormonal Therapy

Hormonal therapy is used after the patient has been tested to determine whether estrogen or progesterone receptors are present. Estrogen receptor (ER-positive) cancers and progesterone (PR-positive) cancers are more likely to respond to hormonal therapy.

Radiation Therapy

Radiation therapy may be used in conjunction with those therapies noted above or alone. Sometimes radiation therapy is used before surgery to shrink the size of the tumor. However, it is more commonly used as a post surgical treatment to aid in destroying cells that may not have been excised.

Breast Cancer Staging

It is important to remember that staging of breast cancer is an important tool used to determine treatment options. Staging is specifically used to gauge the size and extent of the patient's tumor. Many modalities may be used to stage cancer. They include, but are not limited to, MRI, mammography, biopsy, CT, and nuclear medicine. To stage cancer, the American Joint Committee on Cancer places the cancer in letter classifications using the TNM classification system. The letters designate the T (tumor size), N (palpable node), and M (metastasis).

A T label followed by a number 0–4 describes the tumor size and if it has spread. The higher the T number the larger the tumor. The N followed by a number 0–3 indicates the node involvement in the breast. M followed by 0–1 indicates whether the tumor has spread to a distant site.

RECONSTRUCTIVE SURGERIES

Patients may also elect to undergo reconstruction after mastectomy procedures. Methods include breast implants, and traverse rectus abdominis muscle (TRAM) flap and latissimus dorsi muscular tissue reconstruction.

Implants

Implant surgery, as well as any reconstructive surgery, is purely elective. The method of insertion is dependent on anatomy, health of the patient, stage of cancer, and patient preference. The reconstruction may be immediate or delayed. Delayed reconstruction is necessary if the patient is undergoing continued adjuvant therapy or if the patient's skin is too tight to merit an immediate implant procedure. Nipple reconstruction may be completed during the initial procedure or at a later time.

Flap Reconstruction

Flap surgeries use tissue or muscle from other parts of the body to help reconstruct the breast. There are different types of surgery as noted below.

TRAM Flap Reconstruction

TRAM stands for the transverse rectus abdominis muscle, which is located in the lower abdomen, between the waist and the pubic bone. The muscle tissue from

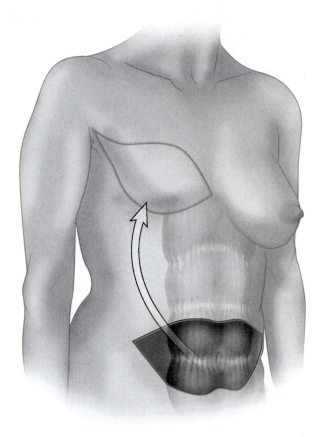

Figure 1–4   TRAM Flap

the abdomen is formed into a breast and sewn in place. The TRAM is very popular, as a "tummy tuck" evolves with the reconstructive process (Figure 1–4).

Latissimus Dorsi Reconstruction

Latissimus dorsi reconstruction, Figure 1–5, uses the muscle from the patient's back to aid in reconstruction of the breast. A tunnel is made under the skin in which an oval section of skin, fat, and a portion of the latissimus dorsi muscle are fed through. Blood vessels are not disturbed as the tissue is made into a breast and sewn into place. Because there is so little body fat in this part of the back, the latissimus dorsi is a good option for a woman with small- to medium-sized breasts.

Arterial Reconstruction

Arterial reconstructions are named for the arteries that supply the blood flow. Some arterial reconstructions include the tissue and vasculature but do not include the musculature. Perforation of the musculature is required,

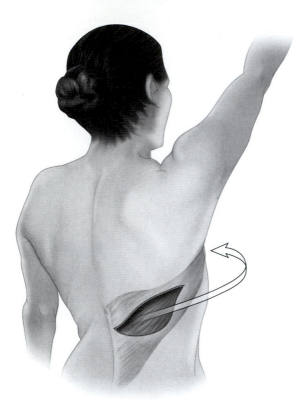

and the tissue and vasculature is moved through the perforation to the reconstructive sight. Options include the DIEP (deep inferior epigastric artery and the deep inferior epigastric vein) and SIEA (superficial inferior epigastric artery flap, which uses small vasculature just beneath the skin surface).

Figure 1–5   Latissimus Dorsi Reconstruction

REVIEW QUESTIONS

Directions: Choose the word or statement that best completes each question.

1. The estimated risk for breast cancer is which of the following?

   A. 1 in 8

   B. 1 in 10

   C. 1 in 12

   D. 1 in 15

2. Which of the following is the greatest single risk factor for breast cancer?

   A. age

   B. gender

   C. age of first menstruation

   D. number of pregnancies

3. The process used to predict a tumor's type and extent of metastasis is which of the following?

   A. staging

   B. screening

   C. testing

   D. localization

4. Which of the following is considered to be a minor risk factor in the development of breast cancer?

   1. family history

   2. advanced age

   3. obesity

   A. 1 only

   B. 2 only

   C. 3 only

   D. 1, 2, and 3

5. Which is a true statement?

   A. Males are nearly as susceptible to breast disease as females

   B. Young women have no risk of breast disease

   C. Cancerous lesions are more common than noncancerous lesions

   D. Increasing age increases the risk of breast cancer

6. Signs and symptoms of breast disease may include which of the following?

   1. breast lump

   2. nipple discharge

   3. skin dimpling

   A. 1 and 2 only

   B. 1 and 3 only

   C. 2 and 3 only

   D. 1, 2, and 3

7. The BSE should be performed at the following intervals:

   A. yearly

   B. monthly

   C. biannually

   D. only when seeing a health professional

8. Treatment options for confirmed breast carcinoma may include all of the following except

   A. lumpectomy

   B. mastectomy

   C. needle aspiration

   D. radiation therapy

9. The American Cancer Society recommends that a yearly mammogram be performed starting at which of the following ages?

   A. 30 years

   B. 40 years

   C. 50 years

   D. 60 years

10. Which of the following questions would be beneficial to the patient history before a mammogram?

    1. prior breast surgery

    2. age of first menarche

    3. number of previous pregnancies

    A. 1 only

    B. 2 only

    C. 3 only

    D. All of the above

11. Which of the following are (is) of most concern when documenting family history?

    A. breast cancer in a parent

    B. breast cancer in a grandparent

    C. breast cancer in a relative

    D. all of the above

12. Which of the following is a primary tool for secondary diagnosis?

    A. mammography

    B. ultrasound

    C. MRI

    D. PET

13. A patient with breast cancer in one breast will have _____ risk of developing cancer in the opposite breast.

    A. greater

    B. lesser

    C. about the same

    D. none of the above

14. Which of the following uses a large "gun" type of biopsy instrument?

    A. FNA

    B. needle localization

    C. core biopsy

    D. all of the above

15. The orange peel effect is commonly due to which of the following?

    A. inflammation

    B. nipple discharge

    C. nipple inversion

    D. skin dryness

16. Which of the following is completed by a professional?

    1. BSE

    2. CBE

    3. mammography

    A. 1 and 2 only

    B. 2 and 3 only

    C. 1 and 3 only

    D. all are completed by a professional

17. Which of the following may increase the risk of breast cancer?

    1. childless female

    2. hormone replacement therapy

    3. late menopause

    A. 1 and 2 only

    B. 2 and 3 only

    C. 1 and 3 only

    D. all may have an effect

18. Which of the following is a procedure used to identify tissue for the surgeon to surgically remove?

    A. FNA

    B. needle localization

    C. core biopsy

    D. pneumocystography

19. Ductography may be used when which of the following are (is) present?

    A. discharge

    B. blood

    C. fluid

    D. all of the above

20. When conducting the BSE, the woman should do which of the following?

    1. Look at breasts in a mirror

    2. Use the pads of the fingers

    3. Examine breast standing and/or laying down

    A. 1 only

    B. 2 and 3

    C. 1 and 3

    D. All of the above

21. The term benign is used to describe which of the following?

    A. a cancerous lesion

    B. a noncancerous lesion

    C. a stellate structure

    D. a milk ridge or line

22. Which of the following ages should have a clinical breast examination every THREE years?

    A. Women 20–39

    B. Women 40–45

    C. Women 46–50

    D. Women 51–60

23. Which of the following procedures is not utilized in reconstruction of the breast?

    A. SIEA

    B. TRAM

    C. DIEP

    D. TUTP

24. Which of the following are factors when considering treatment options for persons with breast cancer?

    1. Stage of the cancer
    2. Previous biopsy
    3. Age of the patient

    A. 1 and 2
    B. 1 and 3
    C. 2 and 3
    D. All of the above

25. Lymphoscintigraphy is a term which may also be known as which of the following procedures?

    A. Lymphography
    B. Pneumocystography
    C. Sentinel node mapping
    D. Ductography

26. Which of the following procedures are secondary tools used in the diagnosis of suspected breast disease?

    A. MRI
    B. Biopsy
    C. Sentinel node mapping
    D. All of the above are secondary tools used for diagnosis.

27. _____ uses magnification, air and aspiration to reduce a cystic lesion.

    A. MRI
    B. Pneumocystography
    C. Ductography
    D. Sentinel node mapping

28. Of the three basic types of biopsy procedures which is used to evaluate nonpalpable lesions which will likely go to surgery?

    A. FNA
    B. Core biopsy
    C. Needle localization
    D. All of the above

29. Which of the following is not a form of benign breast disease?

    1. radial scar
    2. fibroadenoma
    3. lipoma
    4. lobular carcinoma

    A. 1 and 2
    B. 3 and 4
    C. 4 only
    D. 1 and 4

30. Which of the following would not be a type of breast conservative therapy?

    A. lumpectomy
    B. partial mastectomy
    C. quadrantectomy
    D. total mastectomy

ANSWERS AND RATIONALES

1. **(A)** According to the latest statistics from the American Cancer Society, an average of one in eight women will develop cancer over her lifetime.

2. **(B)** Women are 100 times more likely to develop breast cancer than men. Gender is the number one risk factor for breast cancer.

3. **(A)** Cancer staging systems describe how far cancer has spread anatomically.

4. **(C)** Obesity is considered a MINOR risk factor as diet has been linked to cancer. Family history and age are considered MAJOR risk factors.

5. **(D)** A woman's risk of breast disease constantly increases as she gets older. Most breast cancers are found in post menopausal women.

6. **(D)** Lumps, discharge, erythema, skin dimpling, skin thickening, edema, areola and nipple changes.

7. **(B)** The American Cancer Society encourages women to perform BSE each month on the same date or immediately after her period.

8. **(C)** Needle aspiration may be used to help confirm breast cancer but is not a treatment.

9. **(B)** A baseline mammogram is established for the use of comparing mammography examination and should be done between the ages of 30 and 40 years. Yearly mammography should begin at the age of 40.

10. **(D)** Information that should be included on the patient history form include any prior breast disease, age of first period, number of pregnancies, hormone replacement therapy, any family history of breast cancer, date of last mammogram.

11. **(A)** Breast cancer in a parent is of most concern when documenting family history. First blood family members (mother, daughter, sister) are of most concern. Only about 10% of breast cancers are hereditary.

12. **(B)** Ultrasound is the most commonly used modality to aid in diagnosis of breast anomalies.

13. **(A)** Women who develop cancer in one breast have a much greater risk of developing cancer in the opposite breast.

14. **(C)** Core biopsy uses an 11–14 gauge needle which is placed in a rapid-fire instrument to obtain a sample.

15. **(A)** The "peau d'orange" is usually an indicator of inflammatory carcinoma.

16. **(B)** Both the clinical breast examination and the mammogram should be completed by a trained professional.

17. **(D)** As noted earlier, early menarche, late menopause, HRT, birth control and a history of no pregnancies all are minor risk factors for breast cancer.

18. **(B)** The needle localization is used to localize the nonpalpable mass. The surgeon will then excise the mass.

19. **(D)** Discharge, fluid of any type, color or odor and blood may all be indications for ductography.

20. **(D)** When examining the breast the pads of the first three fingers should be used. The breast should always be examined in a mirror for symmetry and the patient may conduct the BSE upright or supine. It is suggested that both be used.

21. **(B)** The term benign defines a noncancerous lesion.

22. **(A)** For women under the age of 40 the clinical breast exam is suggested every 3 years. For women over the age of 40 the clinical breast exam should be done yearly.

23. **(D)** The traverse rectus abdominis muscle (TRAM) as well as the arterial reconstructions include the tissue and vasculature (DIEP, SIEA). There is no such procedure as the TUTP.

24. **(B)** The factors which affect treatment options include but aren't limited to type of cancer, stage, estrogen reception, is it a recurrent or new cancer, age of patient, and menopausal status.

25. **(C)** The terms used to describe a procedure involving identification of the sentinel node are lymphoscintigraphy and sentinel node mapping.

26. **(D)** MRI, biopsy, sentinel node mapping are secondary tools used to identify anomalies already identified with mammography.

27. **(B)** Pneumocystography is a procedure which uses aspiration of cystic fluid, injection of equal part air and mammographic imaging to interrogate the walls of the cyst.

28. **(C)** Needle localization is a procedure usually preformed on nonpalpable lesions that will be surgically evaluated.

29. (C) The two main forms of breast cancer are lobular and ductal. Cysts, lipoma, fibroadenomas, abscesses, gynecomastia, radial scar, ductal ectasia, and fibrocystic changes are not usually associated with cancer.

30. (D) There are conservative breast surgeries that include lumpectomy, partial mastectomy, and segmental mastectomy. A total mastectomy will remove all the breast tissue and may remove some of the lymph nodes under the arm.

2

Instrumentation and Quality Assurance

INSTRUMENTATION

The interior tube design for mammography is altered from standard radiography tubes, allowing its operation characteristics to produce contrast differences amongst the breast tissue. Tubes should preferably be powered by a high frequency or constant potential generator to ensure minimal voltage ripple, producing a more homogenous beam. Tubes should also operate with rotating anodes to reach higher tube rating capabilities.

Filtration

Filtration is necessary to remove low energy photons from the beam that do not contribute to the overall image, but do contribute to patient dose.

■ Total filtration of 0.5 mm Al equivalent is required by regulation

Filtration is matched to target material to help produce the appropriate beam.
Types of target/filter combinations are

■ Molybdenum target with 0.03 mm molybdenum filtration (common and useful for imaging fibro-fatty breasts)

■ Rhodium target with 0.025 mm rhodium filtration (improves beam penetration and useful when imaging dense breasts)

■ Tungsten targets with K-edge filters such as molybdenum, rhodium, yttrium, aluminum (improves beam penetration in patients with dense breasts)

The tube window, which is part of inherent filtration, is comprised of beryllium rather than glass. Beryllium

allows more characteristic radiation to emerge from the tube, which will enhance the image contrast

■ Tube windows must be comprised of 0.8–1.0 mm of beryllium

Kilovoltage

Kilovoltage is operated at a low range that can be manipulated with incremental settings of 1 kVp. The selected kVp will be dependent on target and filtration combinations, radiologist preference, patient breast thickness, equipment calibration, and film/screen characteristics. Low kVp ranges produce a low energy beam resulting in high contrast and increased dose due to the increased mAs values. High kVp ranges may be useful in penetrating denser breasts and will decrease patient dose as mAs values are lowered, but reduce radiographic contrast due to the Compton effect. Higher contrast images are desirable when differentiating between breast structures. The following kVp range values are recommended for the specific target type:

■ Molybdenum targets utilize 24–30 kVp

■ Rhodium targets utilize 26–32 kVp

■ Tungsten targets utilize 22–26 kVp

Heel Effect and Anode Angle

The strongest intensity of the X-ray beam is toward the cathode and therefore the thickest portion of the breast (base) is positioned toward the cathode end of the tube. The cathode is positioned towards the chest wall and with the design of the tube tilt, the central ray aligns parallel with the chest wall. This ensures no breast tissue is missed. The intensity of the beam diminishes towards the anode side of the tube, which is where the nipple is positioned (Figure 2–1). The anode heel effect is more pronounced due to implementation of a shortened SID. This is desired, as a more uniform density is produced among the breast tissue thickness differences.

Focal spot size influences image resolution. The actual focal spot is the point on the anode in which the electrons strike. The effective focal spot is the beam directed towards the patient.

- 0.4 mm or smaller is recommended for routine mammography (0.3 tends to be routine)
- 0.15 mm or smaller is recommended for magnification work

The anode will be angled and tilted by the manufacturer to aid in better heat distribution and for the creation of a small effective focal spot. With the line focus principle design, a larger stream of electrons can be applied (mA) and the smallest effective focal spot produced, allowing for the best image resolution (Figure 2–2).

- 20–22 degrees is the typical anode angle for mammography (A larger anode angle is needed to produce the appropriate field size.)

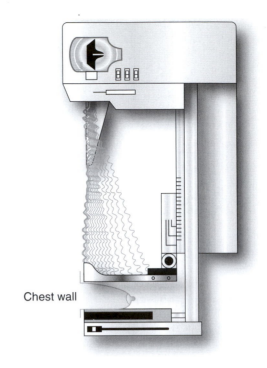

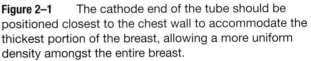

Figure 2–1   The cathode end of the tube should be positioned closest to the chest wall to accommodate the thickest portion of the breast, allowing a more uniform density amongst the entire breast.

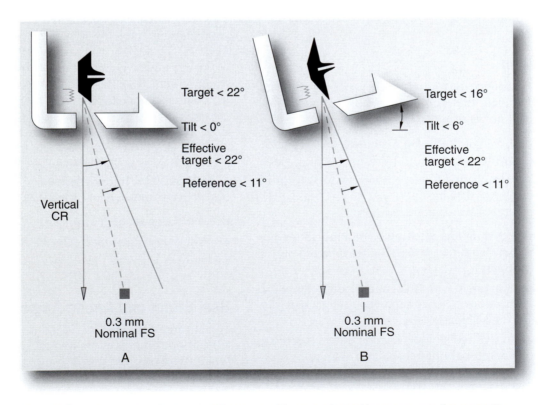

Figure 2–2   By angling the target 22 degrees (A) the projected beam covers the cassette with a shorter distance and focuses the focal spot to the center of the image. By angling the target to only 16 degrees, a smaller focal spot is created and by tilting the tube 6 degrees the anode heating capacity is increased (B).

Automatic Exposure Control (AEC)

Application of AEC provides the greatest level of consistency between exposures and is capable of compensating for numerous breast tissue types. AEC devices found in modern mammography units will either be the ionization chamber or the solid state diode. The AEC capability allows for the detector to be placed in variable positions behind the nipple, depending on the size of the breast and the corresponding densest portion of the breast. Incorrect selection of an AEC cell (for instance, over fatty tissue) may result in underexposure of glandular tissue. AEC systems are required to have a back-up timer to terminate an exposure that has exceeded a pre-selected technique.

Density Settings

Mammography units are equipped with density adjustments that will aid in increasing or decreasing the density based on the breast tissue type being irradiated. To produce optimal density, the density regulator should be applied.

- With each density step, a 0.15 increase or decrease of optical density (OD) should occur.

Image Sharpness

Sharpness of image will be affected by geometric factors such as focal spot size, source to image distance (SID), and object to image distance (OID).

- Focal spot size may be variable depending on imaging requirements for routine work (0.4 or smaller) versus magnification imaging (0.15 or smaller).
- SID tends to be 60–65 cm, but may be variable from 50–85 cm (Figure 2–3).
- OID should be reduced as much as possible to ensure the least amount of unsharpness.

OID at times may be employed for magnification imaging. In these instances, the distance between the breast tissue and the image receptor is increased to enlarge an area of suspicion. Magnification factors of 1.5, 1.6, 1.7, 1.85, and 2 times may be achievable. In order to help compensate for the reduced resolution, application of the smallest focal spot should be utilized. Magnification imaging will reduce resolution due to the increased OID; but with a small focal spot employed, improved visibility of detail is achieved and reduction of scatter radiation reaching the film due to the air-gap technique results.

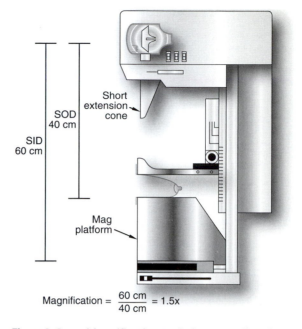

Magnification = $\dfrac{60\ cm}{40\ cm}$ = 1.5x

Figure 2–3 Magnification technique requires the breast to be elevated on a platform to produce a magnification factor. Taking into account the distance and the source to object distance configures the magnification factor.

Image Quality

Image quality can be enhanced through the application of grids, beam limitation devices, and compression. Grids are positioned between the breast bucky support and the image receptor (Figure 2–4).

Grids will assist with the attenuation of primary beam and reduction of scattered radiation to improve overall contrast. Mammographic grids may be linear, focused, or a high transmission cellular grid (HTC). The HTC grid is developed with a criss-cross effect functioning to further reduce scatter (Figure 2–5). Grids prove to increase radiographic quality by removing a majority of scatter effects, but do not decrease the radiation exposure to the breast. Grids are employed for standard imaging and are not necessary for magnification imaging. Magnification mammography will utilize the air-gap technique to reduce the amount of scatter radiation reaching the film thus eliminating the need for a grid.

- Mammography grids may range from 3:1–5:1 (4:1 is typical)
- Mammography grids are of moving type, reciprocating
- Linear grids are constructed with a carbon fiber interspacing at 150–200 lines/inch or 60–80 lines/cm
- HTC grids are constructed of copper strips with air as the interspace material

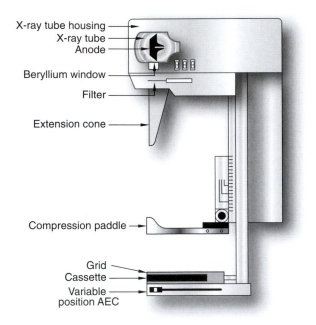

Figure 2–4   Mammography unit with accessory components. Note placement of the grid to be between the breast and the cassette.

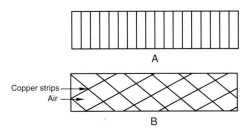

Figure 2–5   (A) represents a standard mammography grid. (B) represents the design of the HTC grid.

Beam limitation devices regulate the size and shape of the X-ray beam and aid in the elimination of scatter. However, in routine mammography the collimated light field must remain the same size as the image receptor, so as not to exclude any tissue on the chest wall edge.

- The collimated light field should not extend beyond the size of the image receptor by more than 2% of the SID

Compression Device

Compression devices on a unit must be designed with a straight chest wall edge and a lip that extends 2–4 cm in height. The lip serves the purpose of preventing chest wall tissue and axillary fat from superimposing on the breast. Compression also serves to decrease the thickness of the breast tissue, making it more uniform (Figure 2–6).

Breast Compression

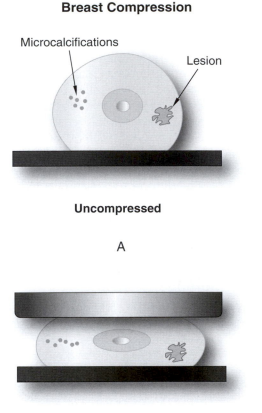

Figure 2–6   Lack of compression (A) increases dose to the patient as the breast is thicker. Lack of compression also fails to spread out structures within the breast and place them closer to the film. Application of compression (B) decreases the thickness of the breast reducing dose to the patient and helps to separate structures apart within the breast, placing them closer to the film.

The compression device must remain parallel to the image receptor when compression is applied. A compression paddle with a flat surface design is seen with mammography units. However, since this design is more apt to compress the thickest region of the breast next to the chest wall, breast tissue towards the nipple may not receive as much compression. Patients may have to experience more discomfort in order to achieve adequate compression towards the nipple. To overcome this, a tilting paddle has been designed to achieve even compression through the thickest region (along the chest wall) and toward the thinner region (the nipple) (Figure 2–7).

Advantages of adequate compression are

- Improved uniform exposure
- Reduced tissue thickness
- Increased visualization of structures

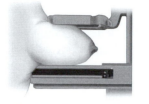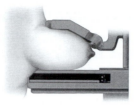

Standard compression paddle   Tilt compression paddle

Figure 2–7   The effects of the newer tilting paddle allows for a more even compression across the entire breast. The tilting paddle continues to apply compression towards the nipple even once appropriate compression has been placed over the thicker base component of the breast.

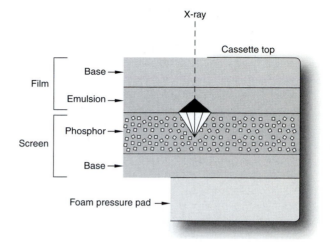

Figure 2–8   Mammography screen and film within a cassette. The single screen design is placed behind the film and in contact with the emulsion side of the film.

- Increased resolution due to decreased structure magnification
- Reduced radiation exposure to the breast tissue

ANALOG IMAGE RECORDING SYSTEMS

Systems for mammography are designed with a slow single speed screen with single emulsion film to acquire high resolution images. A single screen design coupled with a single emulsion film provides for maximum detail or spatial resolution. With this system set-up, a longer processing time is necessary to achieve optimum image contrast. Extended processing increases the amount of time the film is within the developer solution. Furthermore, extended processing could be used to acquire high contrast images and decrease radiation dose to the patient. Extended processing, however, has the downside of increased effect of noise and therefore decreased resolution. The single emulsion mammography film contains a thicker layer of emulsion than compared to dual emulsion film. The emulsion contains the silver halide crystals while the opposite side contains an antihalation layer to improve film resolution by preventing back scatter to the film (Figure 2–8). The single emulsion layer of the film is positioned in front of the screen. Film cassettes containing these components may be of 8 x 10 and 10 x 12 in size. Cassettes should be durable in design of either plastic or carbon fiber, and provide good film screen contact and a light tight environment.

PROCESSING

Automatic processors are complex systems requiring daily monitoring, regular preventative maintenance checks, and scheduled cleanings to ensure optimal performance of the processor. In addition, processor failure, artifacts, and poorly archived films can be minimized. Processor quality control requires the use of a clinical thermometer, sensitometer, densitometer, and a control box of film. The thermometer should not be comprised of glass with mercury in the event that it may break and contaminate the processor. Thermometers should preferably be metal. When assessing solution temperatures, consistency is achieved by acquiring a temperature reading in the same location each time.

Components of Processing

Automatic processing is divided into four steps: developing, fixing, washing, and drying.

- **Developer.** The developer solution will convert the latent image into the manifest image. The developer solution consists of a mixture of different agents to function properly. Maintaining developer temperature is a critical element. Dependent on the manufacturer's specifications, developer temperatures may range from 90–100°F. Regardless, temperatures must not deviate by more than 0.5°F. Increased developer temperatures will alter the speed of the film, resulting in increased film contrast and decreased patient dose. Decreased developer temperatures will slow the speed of the film, requiring increased dose to be administered to the patient to acquire a diagnostic film.

- **Fixer.** The fixer functions to clear any remaining unexposed and underdeveloped silver halide crystals from the film. It also helps complete the development phase and hardens the film. The fixer solution consists of a mixture of different agents as well. However, poorly functioning fixer must be evaluated with a hypo-retention test to ensure long term storage has not been compromised. Temperature control in the fixer cycle is not as critical as it is for the developer. Fixer temperatures will be lower than the set temperature for developer and are allowed to deviate from the recommended temperature by +/– 5°F.

- **Wash Cycle.** This division of processing functions to remove any remaining chemical traces from the film to aid in maximizing long term film storage.

- **Drying.** This is the final phase of processing. This final component utilizes forced heated air. Drying temperatures should be set to film manufacturer's recommendations to ensure adequate drying and to avoid film emulsion blistering.

Extended processing has previously been applied for mammography practice. It is not a common practice today. Extended processing will increase the time the film is immersed within the developer solution to acquire a high contrast film. The disadvantage of extended processing is increasing the likelihood of film fog (Figure 2–9). However, most mammography

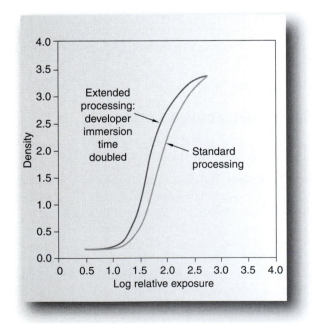

Figure 2–9   Characteristic curve showing the differences between standard processing and the effects of extended processing.

film manufactured today has inherently higher contrast, allowing for standard processing conditions to be applied.

Sensitometric Curves

Sensitometric curves may also be referred to as $D_{\log}E$ curve, H and D curve, or the characteristic curve. This curve serves as graphical representation of the film's response to the set exposure factors and processing conditions. The curve can be divided into 5 components that contribute to the formation of the overall image (Figure 2–10).

- Base plus fog (B+F) consists of inherent film densities from manufacturing and intrinsic fog. The B+F may also be referred to as minimum density. The age of a box of film or improper film storage may lead to increased B+F.

- Toe is the portion of the curve produced by the phenidone agent. This portion of the curve represents the lightest densities which correlate to the denser structures in the breast.

- Straight line portion represents the useful densities of the film that contribute to the image. It represents densities between 0.5 and 2.5. The straight line portion is graphed in a linear fashion. It is this portion of the curve in which the speed of the film can be assessed along with contrast. Film contrast is represented by the steepness of the slope. A steeper slope indicates a higher contrast, therefore lessening the latitude. Latitude is simply the combination of technical factors that can be used to achieve a selected density range. High contrast is preferred for mammography. On the other hand, a more gradual slope indicates a lower contrast, but increased latitude. This means there would be a greater number of technical factor combinations possible to achieve the same densities.

- Shoulder is the portion of the curve produced by the hydroquinone agent. This region of the curve represents dark densities which correlate to less dense tissues in the breast.

- D maximum is the point on the curve in which maximum density is recorded on the film.

DIGITAL IMAGE RECORDING SYSTEMS

The newest alternative to film-screen mammography is the application of full field digital imaging. As it is somewhat difficult to record the wide range of densities emitted by the breast tissue with film-screen

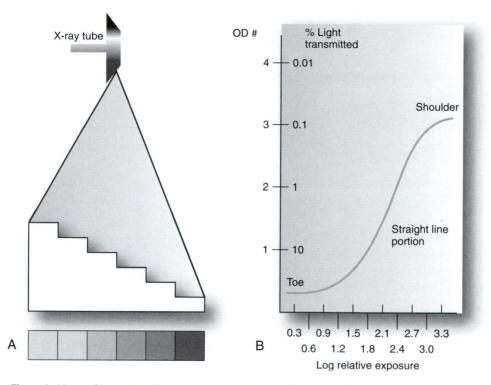

Figure 2–10   Characteristic curve demonstrating divisions of the curve being the toe, straight line portion, and shoulder.

imaging, digital imaging is sought to overcome this. Digital imaging has a wider latitude and represents the variety of breast tissue differences well. Digital imaging plots the values of the intensities detected in a linear fashion, unlike traditional film screen imaging which represents only a certain range of densities for contrast and loses contrast due to over- and underexposure (Figure 2–11).

Digital imaging is advantageous because it allows for grid and nongrid imaging, image manipulation, and portability. Digital imaging systems may be either full field digital mammography (FFDM) or computed mammography (CR). FFDM units operate by replacing film-screen receptors with a detector that will convert X-ray into light which is then converted into a digital signal. There are a variety of detectors that are being utilized by different manufacturers, such as the Phosphor Flat Panel, Phosphor CCD Panel, or the Selenium Flat Panel. A list of approved FFDM units can be accessed on the web at http://www.fda.gov. Computed radiography utilizes phosphor screens within cassettes to capture the image which is converted to a digital image when the phosphor screen is exposed to a laser beam and creates an electrical signal. During this process, electrons will release light photons in proportion to the radiation absorbed by the phosphor. The image reader transmits images to its designated laser printer (Figure 2–12). A laser printer serves as a means to produce a hard copy version of the

mammographic projections without the need for a processor and darkroom.

The digital image contains packaged information, pixels, arranged in columns and rows. An image is constructed in a grid format of columns and rows

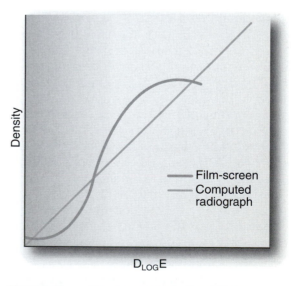

Figure 2–11   Figure represents the differences between film screen imaging and application of digital imaging systems. Digital systems produce a linear response removing the toe and shoulder regions unlike film screen imaging systems.

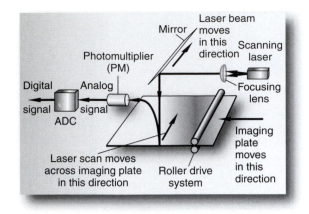

Figure 2–12   The phosphor plate is removed from the cassette and transported through an internal system that passes by a laser. The laser scans the surface of the phosphor plate and releases intensities equal to the radiation absorbed. The analog signal is converted to a digital signal which is transmitted for computer display.

referred to as the image matrix. Each box on the grid defines a pixel. A pixel is assigned with color levels of gray, black, or white, representing the value assigned. Pixels are assigned a bit value that will range between 0 and 2056. Higher pixel bit values represent more brightness. Pixel size is also of importance, as smaller pixel size will increase image detail. As the image is comprised of number values throughout the image matrix, these numbers could be electronically adjusted to enhance the overall image and/or to improve overall visibility within the breast. Viewing the image on the workstation monitor is referred to as soft copy display. Images displayed on the monitor can be altered in brightness and contrast. The process of altering the image is a post processing element referred to as "windowing." During the process of adjusting the image quality factors, ambient light should be controlled to allow for proper post-processing adjustments without compromising the image. Images can also be rotated, inverted, or magnified. There are a variety of monitors appropriate for mammography viewing that are capable of providing high levels of brightness and a wide viewing angle. Cathode ray tube (CRT) was the initial soft copy display appropriate for digital mammography. Since then the field emission display (FED), the liquid crystal display (LCD), and the organic light emitting diode display (OLED) have been developed.

Properties of digital imaging are

- Spatial resolution – The ability to display two points closely related to one another as two separate objects.

- Contrast resolution – The number of shades of gray that can be captured by the detector.

- Dynamic range (latitude) – The range of intensities detected and represented by the signal.

- "S" number or exposure index – A numerical value assigned from the overall exposure and should fall within a range designated by the system. This value helps determine adequate exposure, overexposure, or underexposure. Quantum mottle often co-exists as a result of underexposure. "S" numbers that fall below the assigned range indicate overexposure and those that fall above the assigned range indicate underexposure. In terms of an exposure index, a numerical value falling below the assigned range represents underexposure and a numerical value falling above the assigned range represents overexposure. Different systems may utilize other terminology besides "S" number to define their exposure. The relationship of exposure may be inversely or directly related as described above.

Computer Aided Detection Systems

Computer aided detection systems (CAD) have increased in popularity to serve as a double read system. CAD programs are designed to interrogate the mammogram and flag areas of its noted concern to the radiologist. The radiologist can compare the initial findings to the areas flagged by the CAD system to help reduce the number of pathologies missed. In order for mammograms to be analyzed by the CAD system, a digital image must be produced, which is easily available with FFDM. If a facility does not operate with FFDM, hard copy films can be converted into a digital format by means of a film digitizer.

Digital QC

Similar to film screen mammography, quality control tests are also required with digital systems to ensure proper functioning of the unit. However, specifics on QC testing come forth from the unit manufacturer and the medical physicist, as each unit may vary in its QC requirements. Full-field digital mammography QC duties to be completed by the mammographer may be divided into daily, weekly, monthly, quarterly, and semi-annually. As with film screen mammography, the results of the QC tests should be compared to established criteria and corrective action implemented if necessary.

QUALITY ASSURANCE

Prior to the implementation of the Mammography Quality Standards Act (MQSA), the American College of Radiology (ACR) created a voluntary program of accreditation for mammography facilities. The ACR accreditation program examines equipment, films, image quality, processing, and personnel. In 1992, ACR first published guidelines for implementation of a successful quality assurance program necessary for ACR accreditation. The Mammography Quality Standards Act enacted in 1992 has established quality control and assurance guidelines to ensure quality mammography practices and standardization of facilities. Facilities certified by the FDA are required to undergo annual inspection of their quality assurance programs, including review of quality assurance records and an on-site inspection. Mammography facilities must have obtained accreditation or fall under provisional certification in order to legally offer mammography services. Facilities must contact one of four current accrediting bodies authorized by the FDA: the ACR, the State of Iowa, the State of Texas, or the State of Arkansas. State accrediting bodies may only accredit facilities in their respective state. FDA certification is granted for 3 years and renewal is required before certificate expiration. Certificates of accreditation are recommended for display in a patient visible area, i.e., patient waiting room.

Personnel Requirements

Technologists performing mammography must be licensed to perform general radiographic procedures, and have the initial mammography training (40 hours of documented coursework), initial mammography experience, and then continuing experience (200 mammograms within 24 months), and continuing education (15 CEUs every 3 years) as defined by MQSA. Personnel qualifications also extend to include the medical physicist and interpreting physicians. Medical physicists must be licensed or approved or be certified by the American Board of Radiology or the American Board of Medical Physics. In addition, to meet the initial qualifications of the final regulations they must possess a master's degree or higher in physical science, have 20 hours of physics, 20 contact hours of training in mammography facility surveying, and experience of surveying 10 units. In addition, continuing experience requires inspection of two facilities and six units within 24 months along with 15 CEUs every 3 years.

Consumer Requirements

Mammography facilities are required to establish a consumer complaint mechanism in which the consumers can file a complaint with the facility's accrediting body if the facility is unable to resolve a patient concern or issue.

Medical Audit

Facilities must maintain a medical outcomes audit to track positive mammography results ("Suspicious" or "Highly suggestive of malignancy" category) and correlate it to the pathologists' investigative result. This audit system may be maintained in a logged format by paper or computer. The system must include a method in which pathology results are acquired and correlated with interpreted positive case findings. Documentation of the audit review is required by the interpreting physician. The medical audit system is reviewed on an annual basis and is useful in determining facility false positive or false negative rates.

Record Keeping

Patient films and medical records must be maintained for a minimum of 5 years. However, in instances when a patient has no other mammographic studies at that facility, the patient films and medical record must be maintained for a minimum of 10 years. Some states may have laws requiring this information to be maintained for a longer period of time.

Patient Reports

Mammographic reports must include the name of the patient, an alternate identifier such as a number, date of the patient's exam, the interpreting radiologist's name, and mammographic findings, according to the MQSA assessment categories.

Assessment Categories

The ACR has developed a standardized reporting system known as the BIRAD (Breast Imaging Reporting and Data) system to guide physicians for the coding and assessment of breast cancer. This system is widely used by physicians and surgeons nationwide. The BIRAD assessment categories are as follows:

- Category 0 – Need additional imaging evaluation and/or prior mammograms for comparison.
- Category 1 – Negative
- Category 2 – Benign findings
- Category 3 – Probably benign finding—Initial short term follow-up suggested
- Category 4 – Suspicious abnormality—Biopsy should be considered
- Category 5 – Highly suggestive of malignancy—Appropriate action should be taken
- Category 6 – Known biopsy—Proven malignancy—Appropriate action should be taken

MQSA has also developed assessment categories, but the ACR categories were in existence prior to the final regulations of the MQSA. The MQSA categories, like the ACR categories, were developed with the intent of minimizing the confusion with mammography interpretation and reporting. All mammography reports must identify at least one assessment category from either MQSA or ACR BIRADS. The MQSA assessment categories are as follows:

- Negative
- Benign – Negative assessment
- Probably Benign – High probability of a benign finding, but a short term follow-up is suggested
- Suspicious – Indicates a definite probability of being malignant
- Highly Suggestive of Malignancy
- Known Biopsy Proven Malignant
- Incomplete – Additional imaging or comparison mammogram necessary

Communication of Patient Results

Communication of patient results must be in a written format in terminology a patient can understand. Results must be relayed to the patient within 30 days of the mammographic procedure. Patient results must also be communicated to the patient's ordering physician as well. Patient exam results that are classified as "Suspicious" or "Highly Suggestive of Malignancy" should result in an immediate contact with the patient. It is suggested by the FDA that patient communication should occur within 5 days and to the ordering physician within 3 days. Patient results that fall within the "Incomplete" category of assessment should be conveyed to the patient as soon as possible to schedule additional patient work-up.

Technologist Equipment Quality Control

Processor QC

Purpose: To ensure processor and chemistry consistency for film archival

Frequency: Performed daily before the start of patients

Equipment: Twenty-one step sensitometer and densitometer

Performance Criteria: Mid-density (MD) and density difference (DD) should fall within +/− 0.10 of established baseline. A control value of +/− 0.15

cannot be exceeded. B+F (base plus fog) must fall within +/− 0.03.

Analysis: MD, DD, and B+F must fall within the assigned limits to ensure proper functioning of the processor. If in the event the MD and DD fall outside of +/− 0.10 but are within +/− 0.15, the test should immediately be repeated to rule out human error. Furthermore, if MD and DD fall outside of the +/− 0.15 control limit, the problem must be isolated and corrected before its use in clinical practice. In the event that B+F readings fall outside of the +/− 0.03 control limit, corrective action must be implemented immediately.

Record Maintenance: QC strips must be retained for 1 month and the QC processor charts must be retained for 1 year.

Darkroom Cleaning

Purpose: Minimize artifacts such as dust that may mimic microcalcifications

Frequency: Daily

Equipment: Wet mop, lint free towels

Analysis: Cleanliness of the darkroom is best evaluated through screen cleanliness.

Phantom Imaging

Purpose: To ensure that optimal image density, contrast, uniformity, and image quality are achieved

Frequency: Weekly

Equipment: A square acrylic block equivalent to a 4–4.5 cm breast with a round acrylic disc secured to its surface so as not to obscure simulated internal phantom structures

Control Limits: Phantom image should be viewed by the same person, on the same viewing station, and at the same time of day. Phantom images should evidence at least four fibers, three speck groups, and three masses

Analysis: Film density should be greater than 1.2 with a control limit of +/− 0.20. A density difference should be at least 0.40 with a control limit of +/− 0.05 for the 4 mm disk. Each phantom must be scored and add up to a minimum of 10 points.

Record Maintenance: Retain records for entire year.

Screen Cleaning

Purpose: To remove dust and dirt from screens

Frequency: Weekly or any time when necessary

Equipment: Screen cleaner, canned air, or lint free wipes (follow manufacturer's instructions)

Analysis: Following screen cleaning, mammographic images will evaluate the effectiveness. Screens should be individually numbered for identification.

Viewbox Uniformity

Purpose: To ensure consistent and optimal viewing conditions

Frequency: Weekly

Equipment: Glass cleaner and towel

Analysis: Viewbox bulbs should be evaluated for uniformity and all bulbs should be replaced simultaneously. The luminance for a mammography viewbox should register 3500 nit with a light meter.

Visual Checklist

Purpose: To ensure mammographic equipment is working properly

Frequency: Monthly

Equipment: Checklist

Analysis: Any item on the checklist that fails to meet the passing criteria should either be replaced or serviced for correction.

Repeat Analysis

Purpose: To determine the total number of repeats and to isolate causes of repeats

Frequency: Monthly (if a volume of 250 is achieved) or quarterly as per the ACR 1999 Guidelines

Equipment: A means to determine the repeat rate and reject rate. Total percentage of repeats = total # of rejected films/total # of films exposed. Percentages of repeats per category = total number repeats in the category/total repeats for all categories.

Control Limit: 2% or less is ideal but calculations less than 5% are acceptable

Analysis: At least 250 patients are recommended for a valid analysis.

Fixer Retention

Purpose: To ensure proper processing conditions for film archival purposes

Frequency: Quarterly

Equipment: Hypo Test Kit and unexposed film

Control Limit: Less than 5 μg/cm^2 (compare with hypo estimator strip)

Analysis: Test results that are not within the guidelines require the test to be immediately repeated, and if similar results are obtained, corrective action is necessary. Corrective action may include checking water levels in the wash tank, ensuring the wash water flow rate is set to the guidelines of the manufacturer, or checking the fixer replenishment rate.

Darkroom Fog

Purpose: To ensure white light or safelight leaks are not contributing to film fog

Frequency: Semi-annually

Equipment: Phantom, densitometer, opaque card, and a timer

Control Limit: Density difference obtained should be no greater than 0.05

Analysis: The density difference obtained from the adjacent comparison of the fogged portion to the unfogged portion should not be greater than 0.05. If the value is greater than 0.05, there is a source of fog that must be determined. The darkroom should be evaluated for light leaks and imperfections to the safelight.

Film Screen Contact

Purpose: To ensure adequate film screen contact to achieve maximum image sharpness

Frequency: Semi-annually

Equipment: 40 wires/inch mesh positioned between acrylic sheets, loaded cassettes, and a densitometer

Control Limits: Films with areas of irregularity greater than 1 cm should be retested before discarding the cassette/screen. Films with multiple areas of increased density, but each area measuring less than 1 cm, are considered acceptable.

Analysis: Films with areas of increased density measuring more than 1 cm should first undergo retesting. This involves recleaning the screen/cassette, reloading, reexposing, and reevaluating. If the problem isn't resolved by this process, the cassette must be removed from clinical practice. Films that present with five or more areas of increased density, which measure less than 1 cm diameter, are within acceptable limits. Density readings may represent dirt or dust, damaged cassettes, deteriorated foam within the cassette, or trapped air.

Compression

Purpose: To ensure equipment can adequately apply even compression in both power and manual modes

Frequency: Semi-annually

Equipment: Scale and towels or dedicated compression tool

Control Limits: Manual and power modes must achieve a range of 25–47 pounds

Analysis: Both of the testing modes must attain the above criteria. If not, internal adjustments must be made by the service engineer.

Medical Physicist Quality Control

Annually, medical physicists are required to perform the following tests and implement corrective action either within 30 days of the testing date or immediately:

- Mammographic Unit Assembly Evaluation – The evaluation ensures all the mechanical parts of the unit properly operate. The evaluation extends to include the exposure technique chart. Report within 30 days.

- Collimation Assessment – This assessment determines proper alignment of the X-ray field and the collimated light field. Report within 30 days.

- Evaluation of System Resolution – This test evaluates the focal spot, resolution, and the selected film-screen combination. Focal spot assessment requires the use of a slit or pinhole camera. Report within 30 days.

- AEC System Performance – The evaluation of this system is essential to ensure consistency in image optical density. The system should be capable of optical densities within +/– 0.15 amongst a variable thickness. Report within 30 days.

- Uniformity of Screen Speed – Requires all screens to be evaluated in the cassettes. Upon comparison, the OD should not vary by more than 0.30, ensuring consistent OD attainment. Report within 30 days.

- Artifact Evaluation – Processing artifacts, film handling and storage artifacts, and exposure artifacts are examined. Report within 30 days.

- kVp Accuracy and Reproducibility – The test is designed to ensure that the unit is accurate within +/– 5 % of the pre-selected kVp value and should be reproducible with less than 0.02 variation. Report within 30 days.

- Beam Quality Assessment – The test evaluates and ensures that the half-value layer (HVL) of the X-ray beam is able to penetrate the breast tissue, produce adequate contrast, and reduce patient exposure to the breast. Report within 30 days.

- Breast Exposure and AEC Reproducibility – Breast entrance exposure is tested with the utilization of a breast phantom with 50:50 distribution of glandular to fatty tissue in a 4.2 cm compressed breast. AEC reproducibility aims to ensure that consistent optical densities are achievable regardless of breast thickness or tissue type. Report within 30 days.

ACR Recommended and Required MQSA Quality Control Tests for Technologists

QC Test	MQSA Required	Frequency	Corrective Action Taken
Darkroom Cleaning	Yes	Daily	
Processor QC	Yes	Daily	Immediate
Screen Cleanliness		Weekly	
Viewboxes & Viewing Conditions		Weekly	
Phantom Images	Yes	Weekly	Immediate
Visual Inspection		Monthly	
Repeat Analysis	Yes	Monthly OR Quarterly	Within 30 days of test date
Fixer Retention	Yes	Quarterly	Within 30 days of test date
Darkroom Fog	Yes	Semi-annually	Immediate
Screen-Film Contact	Yes	Semi-annually	Immediate
Compression	Yes	Semi-annually	Immediate

- Radiation Output Rate – This test ensures that a mammography unit is capable of producing the minimum output values when operating at 28 kVp. Report within 30 days.

- Measurement of Viewbox Luminance and Room Illuminance – This test ensures that mammography viewboxes produce a luminance of 3500 nit and room illuminance of 50 lux or less. Report within 30 days.

- Average Glandular Dose – This dose is calculated with the use of a FDA approved phantom. The entrance exposure and the HVL for the kVp value is utilized for the calculation and then compared to the chart to determine operation within limits. Report immediately.

- Image Quality Evaluation – This test evaluates the entire imaging chain from the production of the film, the image receptor, processing and viewing conditions, and observing for any deviations in image quality. Report immediately.

REVIEW QUESTIONS

Directions: Choose the word or statement that best completes each question.

1. The base of the breast should be positioned
   A. at the anode end of the image receptor
   B. at the cathode end of the image receptor
   C. Doesn't apply as the breast is evenly compressed
   D. None of the above

2. Beryllium windows are preferred for mammography over glass windows because beryllium
   A. hardens the beam, improving subject contrast
   B. softens the beam, improving subject contrast
   C. decreases patient dose
   D. increases patient dose

3. The purpose of filtration in mammography is
   A. to remove the high energy photons from the beam
   B. to remove the mid energy photons from the beam
   C. to remove the lowest energy photons from the beam
   D. more than one of the above

4. The point on the anode in which the electron stream hits is
   A. the actual focal spot
   B. the effective focal spot
   C. the anode angle
   D. the focal spot

5. Which of the following does not describe a benefit of adequate compression of the breast?
   A. Reduced geometric unsharpness
   B. Decreased image contrast
   C. Reduced glandular dose
   D. Enhanced image contrast

6. Which of the following criteria for a compression device do not apply?
   A. The compression device must remain parallel to the image receptor
   B. The compression device must match the size of the image receptor for standard imaging
   C. The compression device is designed with a 3 cm in height lip
   D. The compression device is designed with a curved chest edge wall

7. To overcome poor image resolution, which of the following should be applied?
   A. The smallest focal spot
   B. The largest focal spot
   C. Increased OID
   D. Increased SID

8. Magnification imaging typically involves
   A. 3:1 grid
   B. 4:1 grid
   C. 5:1 grid
   D. no grid

9. A category of 0–6 assigned and noted on a patient report represents the
   A. medical audit outcomes
   B. consumer complaint mechanism
   C. BIRAD assessment
   D. physicist findings

10. Which of the following factors would be classified as a disadvantage for extended processing?
    A. Higher image contrast
    B. Increased patient dose
    C. Film fog
    D. None of the above

11. The area of the toe on the H&D curve represents
    A. darkest density region
    B. breast tissue with highest density
    C. breast tissue with lowest density
    D. overall film contrast

12. Which of the following would be a result of developer temperatures operating below optimal levels?
    A. Increased film speed
    B. Decreased patient dose
    C. Increased patient dose
    D. Increased latitude

13. Which of the following factors would yield the best image?
    1. Single emulsion film
    2. Double emulsion film
    3. Small emulsion crystals
    4. Large emulsion crystals
    A. 1 and 3
    B. 1 and 4
    C. 2 and 3
    D. 2 and 4

14. Film latitude is expressed as _____ in digital imaging.
    A. latitude
    B. dynamic range
    C. a matrix
    D. image contrast resolution

15. Which of the following is a limitation of digital mammography?
    A. Contrast resolution
    B. Spatial resolution
    C. Portability
    D. Dynamic range

16. Applying close collimation to the margins of the breast during routine imaging will affect
    A. image markings
    B. image contrast
    C. image viewing
    D. image resolution

17. Processor QC charts are required by MQSA to be retained for a period of
    A. 30 days
    B. 6 months
    C. 1 year
    D. 3 years

18. To establish initial operating levels for the processor, a QC strip
    A. should be run for 3 days
    B. should be run for 5 days
    C. should be run for 7 days
    D. a baseline can be established on the first day

19. Grids are primarily implemented for mammography to
    A. lower patient dose
    B. increase scatter production
    C. improve resolution
    D. increase contrast

20. Grids recommended for mammography use should be
    A. 4:1
    B. 8:1
    C. 12:1
    D. 15:1

21. Which of the following may result in an increased base plus fog (B+F) measurement?
    1. Aged film
    2. Incorrect safelight bulb wattage
    3. Poor quality image receptor
    A. 1 only
    B. 1 and 2
    C. 2 and 3
    D. all of the above

22. Which phase of processing is most responsible for ensuring long term film archival?
    A. Development
    B. Fixing
    C. Washing
    D. Drying

23. The fixer tank must maintain a temperature that may not deviate beyond the manufacturer's recommendation by
    A. 0.5°F
    B. 5°F
    C. 7°F
    D. 10°F

24. Which of the following QC tests may be utilized to evaluate film archival and processing conditions?
    1. Phantom imaging
    2. Processor sensitometry
    3. Fixer retention
    A. 1 and 2
    B. 2 and 3
    C. 1 and 3
    D. all of the above

25. Poor film screen contact would appear on a film as
    A. no change in density
    B. increased density
    C. decreased density
    D. no density

26. The lip of the compression paddle should be designed with which of the following?
    1. Straight edge chest wall
    2. Curved edge chest wall
    3. 2–4 mm lip
    4. 2–4 cm lip
    A. 1 and 3
    B. 2 and 3
    C. 1 and 4
    D. 2 and 4

27. Which of the following describes "extended processing"?
    A. Overall increased immersion time within the processor cycles
    B. Increased immersion time within the developer cycle
    C. Increased immersion time within the fixer cycle
    D. Increased time between when the image was acquired and when the film was processed

28. Which of the following QC tests should be completed quarterly?
    1. Darkroom fog
    2. Fixer retention
    3. Phantom imaging
    A. 1 only
    B. 2 only
    C. 3 only
    D. All of the above

29. The recommended volume of patients for a repeat analysis is
    A. 100
    B. 250
    C. 400
    D. 500

30. When processor QC is being performed and it is noted that the MD (mid density) and the DD (density difference) fall outside of +/− 0.10 control limit, but within the +/− 0.15 control limit, what is the next step taken?
    A. The processor is within limits, patient films can be processed
    B. The processor QC strip should be run again later in the day
    C. The processor QC strip should be run again immediately
    D. The processor should be maintenanced

31. Which of the following describes a high transmission cellular (HTC) grid?
    A. Constructed with a criss-cross effect
    B. Constructed with copper strips and air
    C. Further reduces scatter
    D. All of the above

32. The collimated light field should not extend beyond the edge of the image receptor by more than _____ of the SID.
    A. 3%
    B. 2%
    C. 1%
    D. 0.5%

33. Which of the following is true of digital imaging?
    A. It displays intensity values in a linear fashion
    B. Its intensity values are not lost due to over- or underexposure
    C. It is suited with wide latitude
    D. All of the above

34. An image matrix is defined as
    A. a single pixel
    B. multiple pixels
    C. multiple pixels arranged into columns and rows
    D. multiple pixels arranged into vertical rows

35. A soft copy display of an image
    A. is a printed image
    B. is an image on the computer monitor
    C. is the digital signal
    D. is the digital conversion

36. Altering the brightness and contrast of a digital image is referred to as
    A. pixelating
    B. windowing
    C. pre-processing
    D. image altering

37. The ability to display two points as two separate objects when closely related defines
    A. contrast resolution
    B. windowing
    C. dynamic range
    D. spatial resolution

38. As the pixel size on a digital image decreases, the detail will
    A. increase
    B. decrease
    C. stay the same
    D. none of the above

39. A computed radiography (CR) unit utilizes
    A. an intensifying screen and a scanning laser
    B. a phosphor screen and a scanning laser
    C. a selenium screen and a scanning laser
    D. a photodiode and a scanning laser

40. As the computed radiography (CR) image is exposed to the laser beam, the electrons will release light photons that are _____ the radiation absorbed on the phosphor screen.
    A. greater than
    B. lesser than
    C. equal to
    D. none of the above

41. A patient who has mammographic results that fall within the "Highly Suggestive of Malignancy" category is to have results communicated to them
    A. within 3 days
    B. within 5 days
    C. within 15 days
    D. within 30 days

42. A mechanism in which a patient can file a complaint with the facility's accrediting body is
    A. accreditation complaint mechanism
    B. consumer complaint mechanism
    C. consumer report
    D. patient satisfaction survey

43. A facility is required to maintain a patient's film jacket that has had no other mammographic studies for a minimum of
    A. 3 years
    B. 5 years
    C. 10 years
    D. 15 years

44. The medical audit is performed
    A. to determine the number of "suspicious" or "highly suggestive of malignancy" cases
    B. to determine the overall number of pathology related findings
    C. to figure the number of positive case findings
    D. to correlate the pathology results with the positive findings cases

45. Patient reports must include
    1. mammographic findings
    2. alternate patient identifier
    3. interpreting physician's name
    A. 1 and 2
    B. 1 and 3
    C. 2 and 3
    D. all of the above

46. The BIRAD assessment categories were developed by
    A. FDA
    B. ACR
    C. ART
    D. MQSA

47. Which of the following entities developed systems to assist physicians with a more standardized means of reporting patient results?
    1. MQSA
    2. ACR
    3. ACS
    A. 1 only
    B. 2 only
    C. 1 and 2
    D. all of the above

48. A system in which facility false positive or false negative rates are calculated describes
    A. patient tracking
    B. medical audit
    C. BIRAD assessment
    D. record maintenance

49. Viewbox luminance and room illuminance is required testing by
    A. a mammographer
    B. the QC technologist
    C. the medical physicist
    D. the biomedical engineers

50. The mammography unit assembly is evaluated by the physicist
    A. monthly
    B. quarterly
    C. semi-annually
    D. annually

51. Which of the following provides information regarding image resolution, contrast, and density changes?

    A. repeat analysis

    B. fixer retention

    C. phantom imaging

    D. darkroom fog

52. A minimum of ____ fiber(s) should be visible when scoring an ACR phantom QC test.

    A. one

    B. two

    C. three

    D. four

53. When evaluating a phantom QC test and at least half a fiber in its appropriate location and orientation, the QC technologist should assign this fiber

    A. one-half point

    B. one point

    C. two points

    D. three quarter point

54. Facilities equipped with digital mammography should perform a phantom image

    A. weekly

    B. monthly

    C. quarterly

    D. semi-annually

55. Which of the following are important parameters for QC imaging of a phantom

    1. the same exposure factors applied every time

    2. the same cassette

    3. the imaging cassette must be apart of circulation for patient use

    A. 1 only

    B. 1 and 2

    C. 2 and 3

    D. all of the above

56. According to MQSA guidelines, phantom images must be retained for

    A. 1 month

    B. 6 months

    C. 1 year

    D. 2 years

ANSWERS AND RATIONALES

1. **(B)** The thickest portion of the breast, found closest to the chest wall, should be positioned according to the strongest end of beam intensity, which is the cathode. The intensity of the beam will be weaker at the anode end.

2. **(B)** Beryllium tube windows soften the beam allowing characteristic radiation to emerge from the tube and enhance the contrast of the breast tissue. Glass windows for mammography are not recommended as they will harden the beam and diminish contrast.

3. **(D)** Mammography filtration is recommended to be 0.5 mm Al equivalent. This filtration will remove the lowest energy photons from the beam that do not contribute to image quality, but rather to patient dose and the highest energy photons that will affect the image contrast.

4. **(A)** The actual focal spot is the point at which the electron stream is directed. The effective focal spot is the beam directed towards the patient.

5. **(B)** Adequate compression separates structures of the breast and brings them closer to the image receptor, reduces the possibility of patient motion, reduces radiation dose to the breast as the tissue thickness is decreased, therefore increasing image contrast.

6. **(D)** A compression device must match the size of the image receptor for standard mammographic imaging. A compression device must be designed with a straight chest wall, with a 90 degree lip that extends 2–4 cm in height. The compression device must also function to provide even compression to the breast; therefore, the paddle must remain parallel to the image receptor.

7. **(A)** The smallest focal spot should always be employed to ensure higher image resolution. Routine mammography typically employs focal spot sizes that are 0.4 or smaller and magnification imaging employs 0.15 or smaller. OID should always be reduced as much as possible to bring the structures of the breast closer to the film.

8. **(D)** Grids are not necessary with magnification imaging, as the air-gap technique will reduce the amount of scatter from reaching the film. Grids employed for routine mammography may range from 3:1–5:1, although 4:1 is typical.

9. **(C)** The BIRAD system developed by the ACR is a form of standardized reporting utilized among physicians for coding and assessing breast cancer. The BIRAD system assessment categories are 0–6.

10. **(C)** Extended processing will place the film in the developer solution longer, resulting in higher contrast films and therefore lessening the radiation dose to the patient. Extended processing has disadvantages such as increased chances for film fog and processing artifacts.

11. **(B)** The toe represents the lightest density areas on the curve, corresponding to the densest breast tissue. The straight line portion represents contrast. Mammography film should have a steep slope representing high contrast. The shoulder represents the darkest density areas, corresponding to the low density breast tissues.

12. **(C)** Developer temperatures below set operating levels will require patient dose to be increased to obtain an optimal image. Developer temperatures that are operating above set levels will accommodate the patient with less dose by increasing the speed of the film, but film noise and fog may negatively factor in.

13. **(A)** Single screen cassettes with single emulsion film will provide the best spatial resolution, but will require a longer processing time in order to achieve optimal contrast. Smaller emulsion crystals will also yield the better detail, but lower the speed of the film, requiring increased patient dose.

14. **(B)** Dynamic range replaces the term "latitude" in digital mammography, but has similar meaning. Dynamic range represents the number of intensities that are detected.

15. **(B)** The number of shades of gray that can be captured with digital imaging is referred to as contrast resolution and with digital mammography this is an advantage point, especially for women with extremely dense breasts. Decreased spatial resolution and cost are both disadvantages.

16. **(C)** Mammographic images should be exposed with the light field to extend to the film edges to help mask the breast for better viewing. Image contrast will not improve much with close collimation.

17. **(C)** Processor QC charts are to be retained for 1 year, while the QC strips must be retained for a period of 30 days.

18. **(B)** Processor QC strips should be run for five consecutive days. From the strips obtained, high

density, low density, mid density, and base plus fog should be measured and averages configured to establish initial operative levels.

19. **(D)** Grids for mammography assist with primary beam attenuation and reduce scatter radiation that can be detrimental to film quality. Image contrast is improved with the utilization of grids or implementation of the air-gap technique used with magnification imaging.

20. **(A)** Grids for mammography are typically 4:1, but may range from 3:1–5:1.

21. **(B)** Film is inherently manufactured with dyes or tinting. Elevated B+F levels may be directly related to the age and/or storage of the film or incorrect safelight wattage.

22. **(C)** The fixing phase of the processing cycle is to aid in completion of the development process, remove unexposed and undeveloped crystals, and harden the film. The washing phase is to help remove excess chemicals from the film to prepare for long term storage. Excess chemicals remaining on the film may lead to discoloration. This may be evaluated with the fixer retention quarterly test.

23. **(B)** The temperature of the fixer solution should not deviate above or below the set temperature by 5° F. The developer temperature is more critical to maintain and therefore should not deviate above or below the set temperature by 0.5° F.

24. **(B)** Fixer retention is performed quarterly with the intent to evaluate film archival. However, daily processor QC will also ensure the processor is operating daily within control limits.

25. **(B)** The film screen contact QC test is utilized to ensure the best possible film screen contact to improve detail resolution. Areas of poor film screen contact will appear with an increased density. Increased density areas on the film must not be greater than 1 cm.

26. **(C)** The compression paddle should be designed with a lip of 2–4 cm in height that is straight in design to aid in the prevention of axillary and posterior fat superimposing on the breast tissue.

27. **(B)** Extended processing is when the film is immersed within the developer tank for increased time. The effects of this type of processing are: increased film speed, increased film contrast, reduced patient dose, and possibly decreased film resolution.

28. **(B)** Fixer retention is a quarterly QC test. Phantom imaging is to occur weekly. Darkroom fog, screen film contact, and compression are all tests performed semi-annually.

29. **(B)** The recommended volume of patients is 250 for a valid analysis.

30. **(C)** If the processor QC limits fall outside the +/− 0.10 but under +/− 0.15, the strip should be repeated and reevaluated. If the same results are acquired, the processor should be closely monitored, but patient films can still be processed.

31. **(D)** HTC grid translates into high transmission cellular grid. It is constructed with a criss-cross dispersion of copper strips and air rather than carbon fiber to help further reduce scatter.

32. **(B)** The collimated light field should remain the size of the image receptor so as not to exclude any tissue along the chest wall. The light field should not extend beyond the size of the image receptor by more than 2% of the SID.

33. **(D)** Digital imaging, unlike film screen imaging, offers a wider latitude to represent the various breast densities. The values are displayed in a linear fashion and density values are not lost due to over- or underexposure, as occurs at the toe and shoulder of the characteristic curve of a film screen image.

34. **(C)** An image matrix of a digital image is constructed of multiple pixels arranged into columns and rows. Each box on the grid of the image matrix defines a pixel.

35. **(B)** Soft copy display refers to viewing the image on the computer screen. A hard copy image is the image printed on a piece of film.

36. **(B)** Windowing refers to the alteration of image contrast and brightness.

37. **(D)** A property of digital imaging that displays two points as two separate objects when closely related to one another defines spatial resolution. Contrast resolution is defined as the number of shades of gray that can be captured by the detector. Dynamic range or latitude is the display of a range of intensities.

38. **(A)** As the pixel size decreases on a digital image, the detail increases.

39. **(B)** Computed radiography imaging utilizes a phosphor screen within a cassette to capture an image. The cassette is inserted into an image reader in which a laser beam scans the phosphor screen and creates an electrical signal.

40. **(C)** The laser within the image reader of a CR system functions to free trapped electrons and return them to a state of lower energy. As the

laser beam scans the phosphor screen, the electrons will release light photons that are in proportion or equal to the radiation absorbed.

41. **(B)** If patient exam results are classified as "Suspicious" or "Highly Suggestive of Malignancy," the patient should be contacted within 5 days and the ordering physician within 3 days.

42. **(B)** The FDA requires facilities to have a consumer complaint mechanism in which patients can file a complaint with the facility. If the facility is unable to resolve the issue, the consumer is informed as to how to get in touch with the accreditation body.

43. **(C)** Patient films and medical records must be maintained for a minimum of 5 years. In instances when a patient has no other mammographic studies, patient films and records must be maintained for a minimum of 10 years. Some states may have laws requiring a longer period than 10 years.

44. **(D)** The medical audit system is reviewed on an annual basis and is useful in determining the number of false positive or false negative rates. The audit system correlates the pathology results to the positive findings cases.

45. **(D)** Mammographic reports must include the name of the patient, an alternate patient identifier, date of the exam, interpreting physician's name, and the mammographic findings, according to the MQSA assessment categories.

46. **(B)** The BIRAD Assessment categories were developed by the ACR to provide physicians and surgeons with a standardized means of coding breast cancer.

47. **(C)** Both MQSA and ACR developed categories to create a more standardized environment of patient result reporting. The ACR BIRAD categories were in fact developed before the MQSA assessment categories seen within the final regulations.

48. **(B)** The medical audit, reviewed on an annual basis, is used to determine the number of false positive or false negative rates by correlating patient pathology to positive case findings.

49. **(C)** The medical physicist assumes the responsibility of testing the viewbox luminance and room illuminance annually with a light meter.

50. **(D)** Medical physicists are responsible for evaluating the mammography unit assembly to ensure proper working mechanics annually. The QC technologist may inspect the unit monthly with use of a checklist and is responsible for having the unit serviced if necessary.

51. **(C)** Phantom imaging is an extremely important aspect of a quality assurance program. It provides information regarding image resolution, contrast, density changes, unit output, and potential tube degeneration.

52. **(D)** The phantom imaging QC test requires at a minimum that 4 fibers, 3 speck groups, and 3 masses are visible.

53. **(A)** A whole fiber noted in its correct location is assigned one point. If at least one half of a fiber is visible in its correct location and orientation, then one-half point is assigned for that specific fiber.

54. **(A)** Facilities with digital mammography will abide by the same ACR phantom image requirements as film screen facilities. This means that film screen and digital mammography facilities must perform at least a weekly phantom.

55. **(B)** When performing the phantom QC test, the same exposure factors must be applied each time and recorded. In addition, a designated cassette is used to image the phantom, but is of type that is used for patient imaging. Technical factors applied should be similar to that of clinical imaging. The phantom image should also be processed as a clinical mammogram. A phantom image is performed to evaluate that image quality and contrast are optimal.

56. **(C)** Phantom images must be retained for at least the past full year according to the MQSA requirement.

3

Anatomy, Physiology, and Pathology

ANATOMY

External Appearance

Breast size is genetically determined and is influenced by the percentage of breast tissue to fat tissue within the breast. The breast is positioned on the anterior chest wall just below the second rib or clavicle and extends down to the level of the sixth or seventh rib to form the inframammary fold at the junction with the lower chest wall. Breast tissue also extends from the lateral margin of the sternum to the axilla. The extension of breast tissue from the upper outer quadrant into the axilla is referenced as the Tail of Spence or the axillary tail. The lateral and inferior margins of the breast are considered to be the most mobile borders of the breast.

The nipple represents a point of intersection to divide the breast into four quadrants: upper outer quadrant, lower outer quadrant, lower inner quadrant, and upper inner quadrant. The breast can be further localized by the clock face method and by zones (Figure 3–1). The clock face method positions the hours like a clock face on both breasts. This method of localization may allow pathology to fall at a certain time but correspond to different quadrants depending on the breast in question. For example, the 2:00 position will correlate to the upper inner quadrant in the right breast and the upper outer quadrant in the left breast. A second example, the 3:00 position, would indicate a medial position on the right breast and a lateral position on the left breast. In addition to utilization of the clock face and the quadrant method, the breast can also be referenced by Zone A, Zone B, and Zone C. The designated zone describes the depth of a lesion. Zone A represents the third of the breast that is more superficial, Zone B represents the middle

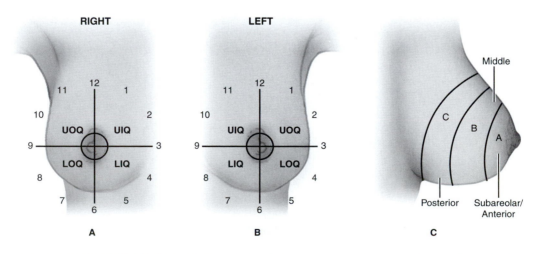

Figure 3–1   (A & B) Four quadrant breast localization and clockface localization method   (C) Zone or region localization referencing depth in the breast

one-third of the breast, and Zone C represents the one-third of the breast closest to the chest wall.

The nipple is surrounded by a region known as the areola, which, on its surface, contains tiny protrusions known as Morgagni's tubercles which are the surface point of the Montgomery's glands. These glands aid in providing lubrication necessary for breast feeding. The region of the areola represents the area where the skin is thinnest (0.5 mm). At the point in which the skin margin meets the anterior chest wall the skin is considered to be its thickest at 2.0 mm. The skin in the region of the breast is anatomically similar to skin elsewhere on the body, containing sweat glands, sebaceous glands, and hair follicles.

Internal Anatomy

The breast tissue is enveloped by layers of connective tissue referred to as fascia. A layer of deep fascia separates the pectoralis muscle from the breast tissue. This deep fascia courses anteriorly beneath the skin surface to encase the mammary stroma. The fascial layer beneath the skin is referred to as the superficial fascia. Breast tissue is given support by a network of fibrous bands known as the Cooper's ligaments that extend from the base of the breast towards the nipple. As Cooper's ligaments lose elasticity or are invaded by a nearby malignancy, an alteration in external appearance will be noted (Figure 3–2 and Figure 3–3).

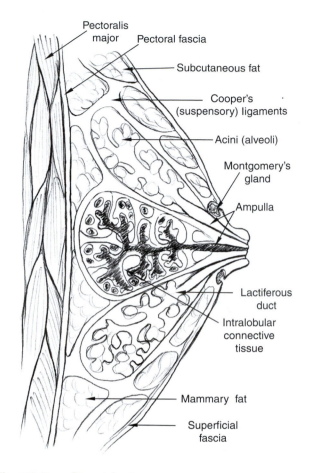

Figure 3–2   Breast Anatomy

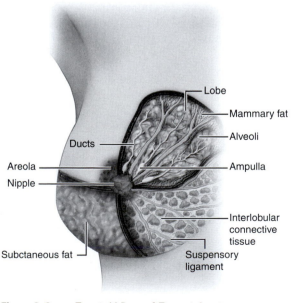

Figure 3–3   Frontal View of Breast Anatomy

The glandular tissue of the breast is arranged in 15–20 lobes that sequence around the breast in a clockwise fashion. In between the glandular lobes lies fibrous and adipose tissue. Each lobe is divided into lobulated segments of tissue that have respective ductal structures that course towards the nipple. Every lobulated segment has a duct that formulates the terminal ductal lobular unit (TDLU). The TDLU is a common site for either benign or malignant pathologies to originate. The TDLU may be subdivided into two components: the intralobular terminal duct and the extralobular terminal duct. The intralobular terminal unit contains the acini or ductules. The intraductal terminal unit lumen is lined with epithelial cells which are surrounded by a layer of myoepithelial cells sporadically positioned around the lumen posterior to the epithelial cells. The myoepithelial cells function to help expel and force the milk towards the nipple during lactation. A basement membrane lies in between the epithelial layers and the surrounding interlobular connective tissue to act as a support mechanism. The intralobular terminal unit communicates with the extralobular unit, forming the entire TDLU, and then anastamose with other ducts as they course towards the nipple. The main lactiferous duct that drains each lobe reaches a point of dilation known as the ampulla before surfacing at the nipple. TDLUs will increase in size and number with pregnancy and lactation. Following the cessation of lactation, the TDLUs will shrink. Towards the progression of menopause, TDLUs continue to atrophy, and eventually the entire breast will be replaced with fatty tissue (Figure 3–4 and Figure 3–5).

Blood Supply and Lymphatic Drainage

The majority of blood supply to the breast is delivered by the internal mammary artery, lateral thoracic artery branches, and intercostal arteries. The majority of drainage for the lymphatic route is towards the axilla and to the internal mammary nodes, but will also include deep system drainage to the infraclavicular and pectoralis nodes. The lymphatic channels drain into the venous system (Figure 3–6).

A typical normal lymph node is oval in shape, 2 cm or less in size, and contains a lucent center.

BREAST PHYSIOLOGY
Cyclic Hormones, Menopause, and HRT

During the proliferative phase of the cycle, which is noted after the menstrual phase until the point of ovulation, estrogen is produced and released by the ovary, and follicular stimulating hormone (FSH) is produced and released by the pituitary gland. These two hormones are preparing the ovarian follicles for the release of an egg at the time of ovulation, and promote ductal proliferation and growth in the breast.

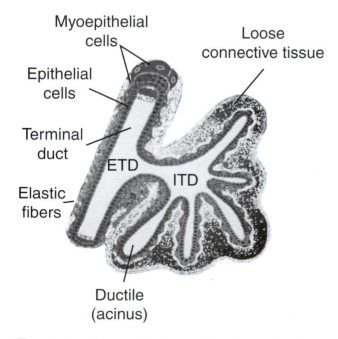

Figure 3–4   Anatomy of a Terminal Duct Lobular Unit (Note: In this figure, ETD represents Extralobular Terminal Duct and ITD represents Intralobular Terminal Duct.)

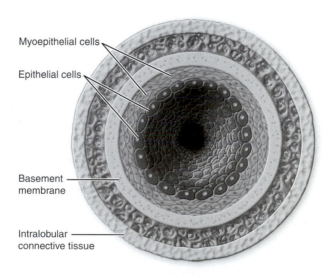

Figure 3–5   Ductal wall cross section demonstrating the location of the epithelial cells, myoepithelial cells, basement membrane, and intralobular connective tissue

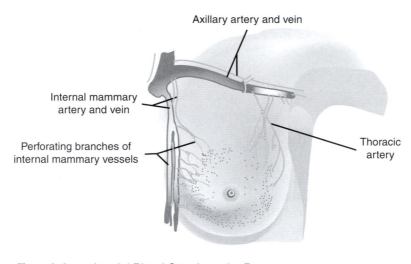

Figure 3–6   Arterial Blood Supply to the Breast

During the secretory phase of the cycle which follows the ovulation event, the progesterone hormone becomes dominant, resulting in thick-ening of the endometrial lining, sustaining the endometrium with embryo implantation, and lobular proliferation and growth. At the end of the secretory phase, approximately day 28, if there is no pregnancy, the progesterone levels fall and the woman will undergo the menstrual phase of her cycle. The endometrium will shed and the tender swollen breasts due to increased interstitial fluids will begin to subside. These repeated cyclic changes during years of menstruation will alter the structure of the breast. It is thought that the greater number of menstrual cycles a woman undergoes, the greater her risk for breast cancer. Once a woman's ovaries cease to function, the breast structures are no longer stimulated and will begin to degenerate and atrophy. This is referred to as involution. The Cooper's ligaments lose elasticity causing the breast to become more pendulous. The glandular tissue begins to atrophy medially and posteriorly and gradually working towards the nipple. The tissue pattern associated with the involution process may be altered with the introduction of hormone replacement therapy (HRT). Women on HRT will experience an increase in the amount of glandular tissue. Women on HRT may mammographically reveal an increased amount of glandular regions within the breast bilaterally. It should be noted of concern when a unilateral region of increased density is seen on the images of patients on HRT, as these women may be at an increased risk of developing breast cancer.

BREAST PATHOLOGY
Pathologic Processes

Abnormalities within the breast will be categorized as either benign or malignant. Mammographic appearance coupled with additional diagnostic tools will aid in disease classification. Underlying breast pathology may also cause surface changes such as alteration in contour, skin redness and/or thickening, and nipple inversion or discharge. Mammographically, the pathology may present with breast tissue asymmetry right to left, breast tissue distortion, masses, and/or calcifications.

Characteristics of Masses

Breast masses may be categorized as benign or malignant dependent upon their mammographic characteristics. Masses are evaluated by their border, density, and tissue make-up.

Border

- Stellate borders appear with irradiating lines off the mass into the surrounding tissue, however the irradiating lines disappear into the lesion's center. This characteristic is suggestive of malignancy. The silhouette sign may appear to have irradiating lines off the mass, but the lines can be followed into and out of the mass, which means the lesion is not truly stellate.

- Smooth or well circumscribed borders are suggestive of benign growth (Figure 3–7).

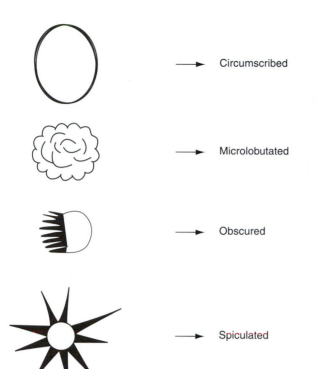

Circumscribed

Microlobutated

Obscured

Spiculated

Figure 3–7   Mass Margin Descriptors

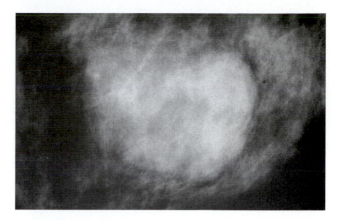

Figure 3–8   Benign Cyst

Density

- Malignancy tends to present with increased density compared to surrounding tissue.

Tissue Make-Up

- Fatty tissue indicates a benign process.
- Fatty and glandular mix usually indicates a benign process.
- Glandular or fibrous make-up indicates a benign or malignant process.

Benign Masses

These are masses that have been categorized as benign disease processes based upon diagnostic and histologic findings.

Cysts

- Fluid accumulation within the ductules (acini) lining the TDLUs causing distention.
- Characterized by being round to oval in shape and well-circumscribed (Figure 3–8).
- Ultrasound may be the modality of choice to determine a truly cystic structure (Figure 3–9).

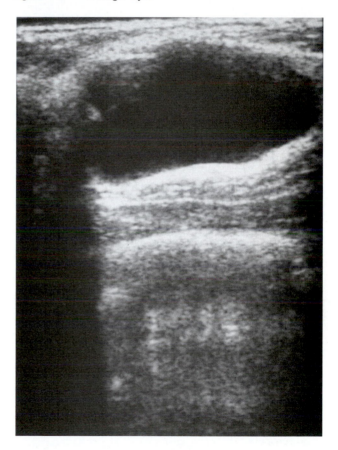

Figure 3–9   Cyst Demonstrated with Ultrasound

Lipoma

- Palpable mass typically located superficially or around the periphery of the breast.
- Appears as a lucent centered mass composed primarily of fatty tissue with encapsulation (Figure 3–10).

Hamartoma

- Encapsulated smooth mass that is an island of glandular tissue due to development variation.

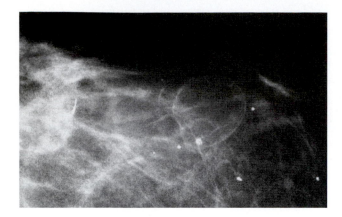

Figure 3–10   Lipoma

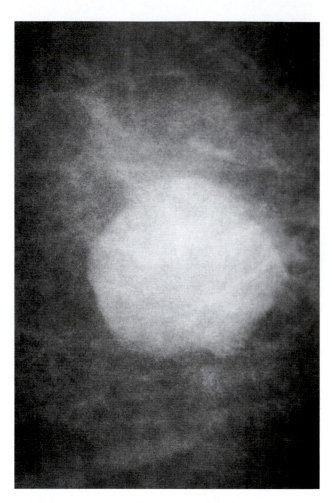

Figure 3–11   Benign Fibroadenoma

Fibroadenoma

- Round to oval well circumscribed mass effect caused by an overgrowth of lobular tissue.
- Common solid mass in younger women which may respond to hormonal changes (Figure 3–11).

Papilloma

- Results from an overgrowth of epithelial cells lining a duct and grows in a cluster like fashion off of a stalk.
- Typically noted in the subareolar region. If it were to grow large enough, the patient may present with nipple discharge.

Radial Scar

- Mammographically it may appear as a mass effect with spiculated (stellate) margins, but has a radiolucent center (Figure 3–12).
- May in fact mimic a malignant lesion, and calls for further diagnostic measures.

Galactocele

- Cysts that form in an obstructed duct that fills with thick, milky fluid during the lactation process or following the cessation of nursing.
- Location tends to be posterior to the areola.

Ductal ectasia

- Result of a duct enlargement around the region of the nipple in middle aged women.
- Associated with nipple discharge if the duct fills with fluid.

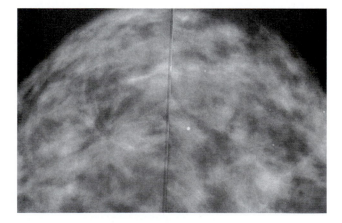

Figure 3–12   Radial Scar

Mastitis

- Bacterial infection of the breast tissues resulting in areas of redness and swelling.
- If infection remains untreated, it could potentially abscess.

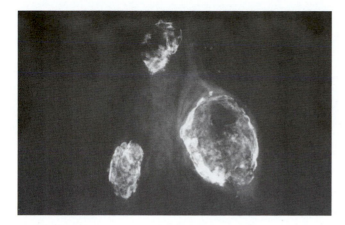

Figure 3–13   Fat Necrosis

Figure 3–14   Intramammary Lymph Node

Other benign findings

■ Hematoma – A result of trauma causing a pooling of blood forming an oval or circular lesion that may calcify over time.

■ Abscess – An area of infection that may present as a reddened and inflamed mass most often noted in the central or subareolar regions of a lactating breast.

■ Fat necrosis – Death of fatty tissue (usually a result of injury) that becomes encapsulated and calcifies with an eggshell appearance. May also be referred to as an oil cyst (Figure 3–13).

■ Lymph nodes – Mammographically visible and are considered normal when visualized with lucent centers and not more than 2 cm in length (Figure 3–14).

Malignant Conditions

Masses can be categorized as malignant disease processes based upon diagnostic and histologic findings.

Features of Malignant Masses

■ Skin thickening

■ Nipple retraction

■ Increased tissue density compared to surrounding tissue

■ Stellate borders– mass appears to radiate out resembling a star

■ Associated with clustered calcifications

■ Breast tissue distortion

■ Could possibly present with a lesser density or well circumscribed margins

■ Nodal enlargement

Inflammatory Carcinoma

■ Rapid growing cancer cells that block the lymphatics of the breast.

■ Symptoms mirror mastitis, but the condition fails to respond to antibiotics.

■ No presentation of a palpable mass.

■ Carcinoma will grow in nest-like fashion within the breast.

■ Rare form of cancer, comprises approximately 1–6% of invasive cancers in caucasian women.

Paget's Disease

■ Form of malignancy at the nipple.

■ Cancer cells will be noted growing into the skin of the nipple.

■ Disease process may be present only at the nipple, or present with disease at the nipple, but also a high probability (50–60%) of an underlying lesion in the breast tissue (Figure 3–15).

■ Associated with redness and crusting of the nipple.

■ Comprises less than 5% of all breast cancers.

Ductal Carcinoma in situ

■ Cancer cell growth is contained within the ducts of a lobe or segment of breast tissue.

■ Ductal calcifications may be evident (Figure 3–16).

Invasive Ductal Carcinoma

■ Cancer type that originates in the duct work of the TDLU which then breaks through the ductal walls and invades surrounding tissues (Figure 3–16).

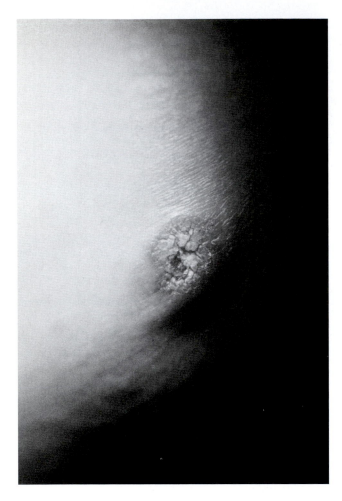

Figure 3–15   Paget's Disease

■ Represents approximately 65% of all breast cancers diagnosed.

Invasive Lobular Carcinoma

■ Cancer type that originates in the lobular epithelium and has the potential to invade into surrounding tissues.

■ Often difficult to distinguish mammographically (Figure 3–17).

Other Malignant Conditions

■ Sarcoma – Rare malignant lesions (account for less than 1%) arising from stromal structures within the breast, i.e., phylloids tumor.

■ Lymphoma – Can occur as a primary lesion or as a migratory metastatic lesion from elsewhere. Accounts for approximately 0.1% of breast cancers. May appear with a discrete intramammary nodule or multiple nodules represented by mammographic density and well circumscribed margins. Axillary lymph nodes may be present with the intramammary nodules.

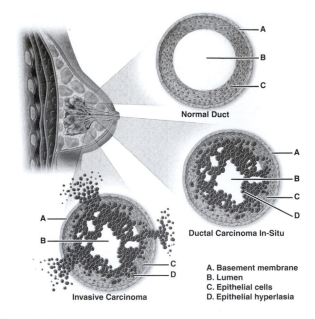

Figure 3–16

A. Basement membrane
B. Lumen
C. Epithelial cells
D. Epithelial hyperlasia

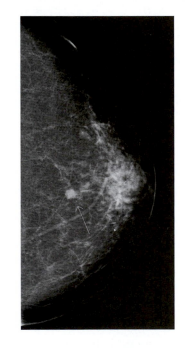

Figure 3–17   Invasive Lobular Carcinoma

Calcifications

Calcifications may present with benign or malignant lesions. Certain characteristics such as shape, size, number, distribution, and associated densities may aid in the differential diagnosis process.

Characteristics of Benign Indicators Calcifications (Figure 3–18):

■ Course or popcorn: Course calcifications due to atrophic fibroadenomas

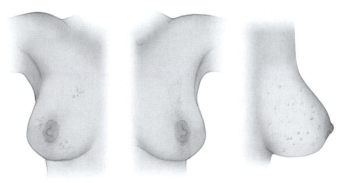

Cluster Type Calcification   Segmental Calcification   Diffuse Calcification

Figure 3–18   Calcification Distribution

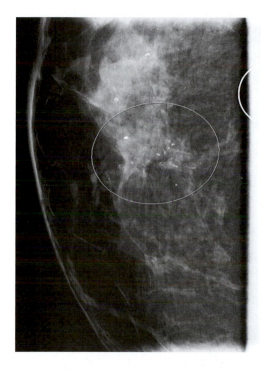

Figure 3–19   Malignant Calcifications

- Rim: Resembles the shell of an egg
- Milk of calcium: Microcysts that present with mixture of fluid and calcified particles. Typically are benign unless noted with other associated findings
- Arterial calcifications: Atherosclerotic process
- Skin calcifications: Round with lucent centers
- Small or large, rod shaped
- Diffuse distribution
- Similar type of calcifications bilaterally
- Calcium deposits positioned within normal appearing breast tissue

Characteristics of Suspicious Indicators of Malignant Calcifications (Figure 3–19):

- Flake shape: Indistinct
- Microcalcifications
- Clusters that increase in number over a period of time
- Irregular size and shape
- Associated density or tissue distortion
- Typically small

REVIEW QUESTIONS

Directions: Choose the word or statement that best completes each question.

1. The skin of the breast is considered to be the thinnest at
   A. the nipple
   B. the base
   C. the Tail of Spence
   D. the areola

2. Breast tissue is positioned on the anterior chest wall
   A. between the 3rd and 7th rib
   B. between the 2nd and 7th rib
   C. just above the clavicle and down to the 5th rib
   D. between the 2nd rib and the inframammary fold

3. The areola surface structures that aid in the release of lubricating fluid are
   A. Cooper's ligaments
   B. nipple
   C. Montgomery's glands
   D. Morgagni's tubercles

4. Which of the following separate the pectoralis muscle from the breast tissue?
   A. Superficial fascia
   B. Cooper's ligaments
   C. Deep fascia
   D. Lymph nodes

5. Cooper's ligaments are
   A. a support network that extends from the medial to lateral aspect of the breast
   B. a support network that extends from the base of the breast to the nipple
   C. a support network that is arranged sporadically through the breast tissue
   D. a support network that is located within the superficial fascia

6. Which of the following may alter the external appearance of the breast?
   1. A malignant invasion into surrounding breast tissues
   2. A macrocalcification
   3. A loss in the elasticity of the Cooper's ligaments
   A. 1 and 2
   B. 1 and 3
   C. 2 and 3
   D. All of the above

7. A 7 o'clock lesion in the right breast may be referenced to which quadrant?
   A. UOQ
   B. LOQ
   C. UIQ
   D. LIQ

8. A common location for either benign or malignant pathologies to originate is
   A. lobe
   B. Montgomery's gland
   C. TDLU
   D. ductal ampulla

9. Which of the following is false regarding the terminal ductal lobular units?
   A. TDLUs will increase in size and number during pregnancy and lactation
   B. TDLUs involute and are eventually replaced by fatty tissue
   C. TDLUs are a site for pathological growth
   D. TDLUs only contain an intralobular terminal unit

10. Which of the following do not contribute to blood supply delivered to the breast?
    A. intercostal arteries
    B. internal mammary arteries
    C. brachiocephalic arteries
    D. lateral thoracic arteries

11. A lesion in the lower outer quadrant of the left breast is located in the
    A. 1 o'clock position
    B. 5 o'clock position
    C. 7 o'clock position
    D. 10 o'clock position

12. Which of the following characterizes a papilloma?
    1. Tends to lie deep within the mammary tissue
    2. May result in nipple discharge
    3. Tends to be benign
    4. Tends to be subareolar in location
    A. 1 and 2
    B. 1, 2, and 3
    C. 2, 3, and 4
    D. 3 and 4

13. Which of the following are associated with malignancy?
    1. Associated clustered microcalcifications
    2. Macrocalcifications
    3. Spiculated edges
    4. Increased tissue density
    A. 1, 2, and 3
    B. 2, 3, and 4
    C. 1, 3, and 4
    D. All of the above

14. Which of the benign pathologies could mimic a malignant one?
    A. Galactocele
    B. Hamartoma
    C. Radial scar
    D. Ductal ectasia

15. Which of the following malignant pathologies fails to present with a palpable mass?
    A. Cystosarcoma Phylloid
    B. Invasive Paget's disease
    C. Inflammatory carcinoma
    D. None of the above

16. A lipoma tends to be
    1. benign
    2. malignant
    3. composed of glandular tissue
    4. composed of fatty tissue
    A. 1 and 3
    B. 2 and 3
    C. 1 and 4
    D. 2 and 4

17. Which of the following may present with a parallel type of calcification?
    1. Atherosclerotic vessels
    2. DCIS
    3. Invasive ductal carcinoma
    4. Ductal ectasia
    A. 1 and 2
    B. 1, 2, and 3
    C. 1, 3, and 4
    D. 2 and 3

18. Which of the following characteristics represent likely benign calcifications?
    A. Irregular size and shape and diffuse distribution
    B. Diffuse distribution, bilateral distribution, and rimmed
    C. Clustered distribution bilaterally
    D. Milk of calcium with associated tissue densities

19. The milk-producing units of the breast are the
    1. acini
    2. ductules
    3. lobes
    A. 1 and 2
    B. 2 and 3
    C. 1 and 3
    D. all of the above

20. The point where the base of the breast intersects with the anterior abdominal wall is the
    A. Tail of Spence
    B. axillary tail
    C. inframammary fold
    D. infraclavicular margin

21. The glandular tissue of the breast may be affected by which of the following factors?
    1. Genetic predisposition
    2. Percentage of body fat
    3. Monthly cyclic changes
    A. 1 and 2
    B. 1 and 3
    C. 2 and 3
    D. All of the above

22. Which of the following physical signs may indicate a potential underlying malignancy?
    1. Recent nipple inversion
    2. A thickened dimpled skin appearance
    3. Nipple discharge
    A. 1 and 2
    B. 2 and 3
    C. 1 and 3
    D. All of the above

23. Which of the following hormones is responsible for lobular proliferation and growth?
    A. Estrogen
    B. Progesterone
    C. Follicular stimulating hormone
    D. Human chorionic gonadotropin

24. The upper outer quadrant of the breast is associated with higher incidence of breast cancer because
    1. it has the highest volume of tissue
    2. it is located closer to the major point of lymphatic drainage
    3. it is the quadrant with the slowest regression of tissue
    A. 1 only
    B. 1 and 2
    C. 1 and 3
    D. all of the above

25. Which of the following calcification presentations may warrant a biopsy?
    1. Associated density
    2. A single punctate calcification
    3. Clustered distribution
    A. 1 and 2
    B. 1 and 3
    C. 2 and 3
    D. all of the above

26. Which of the following would be a likely mammographic appearance of a 60-year-old woman who has been on hormone replacement therapy (HRT) for 5 years?
    A. No change
    B. The breasts may appear with areas of increased fibroglandular tissue
    C. The breasts may appear with dense glandular tissue equally distributed throughout
    D. The breasts may appear with areas of increased adipose tissue

27. A 67-year-old female who is not utilizing hormone replacement therapy (HRT) and who presents with an area of increased density unilaterally would
    A. be of no immediate concern; annual follow-up
    B. indicate the possibility of a pathology presentation
    C. indicate most likely a benign pathology presentation
    D. indicate immediate consultation with radiation oncology

28. What does the zero yield factor mean in mammography?
    A. A negative mammogram
    B. A positive mammogram
    C. The mammogram will not yield many benefits
    D. The mammogram will yield many benefits

29. A lesion is noted within the axillary region of the breast on the MLO view. The lesion appears to be oval in shape with a radiolucent center. This would most likely be
    A. radial scar
    B. fibroadenoma
    C. lipoma
    D. lymph node

30. Which of the following skin visible structures is responsible for the release of lubricating fluid to the region of the areola to accommodate the breast feeding process?
    A. Morgagni's tubercles
    B. Nipple
    C. Lactiferous duct
    D. Montgomery's glands

31. Which of the following pathological processes could be misdiagnosed as a benign occurrence due to its physical presentation of symptoms?
    A. Fibroadenoma
    B. Mastitis
    C. DCIS
    D. Inflammatory breast cancer

32. The suspicious calcifications seen in Figure 3–20 likely represent
    A. macrocalcifications
    B. rim calcifications
    C. DCIS
    D. dermal calcifications

33. Which of the following is depicted by the arrow in Figure 3–21?

    A. TDLU

    B. Intraductal lobular unit

    C. Acinus

    D. Myoepithelial cells

34. A Cooper's ligament would be represented by which letter in Figure 3–22?

    A. A

    B. B

    C. C

    D. D

35. The benign process noted in Figure 3–23 represents

    A. DCIS

    B. papilloma

    C. arterial calcification

    D. rod calcification

36. The image acquired for Figure 3–24, represents which of the following?

    A. clustered microcalcfications

    B. rod like calcifications

    C. macrocalcifications

    D. milk of calcium

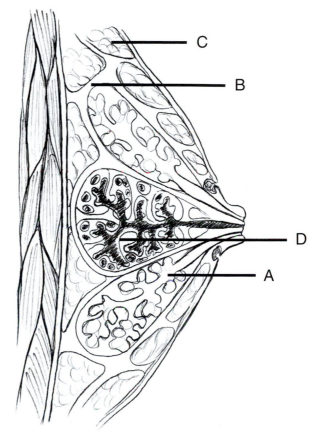

Figure 3–22

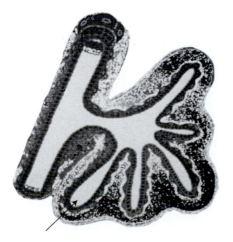

Figure 3–20

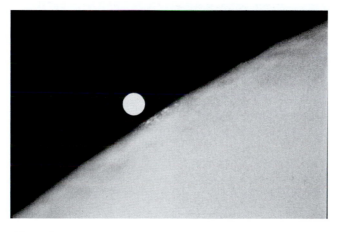

Figure 3–21

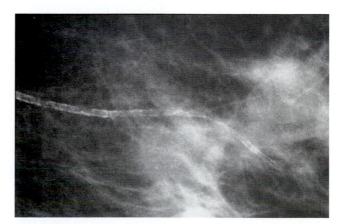

Figure 3–23

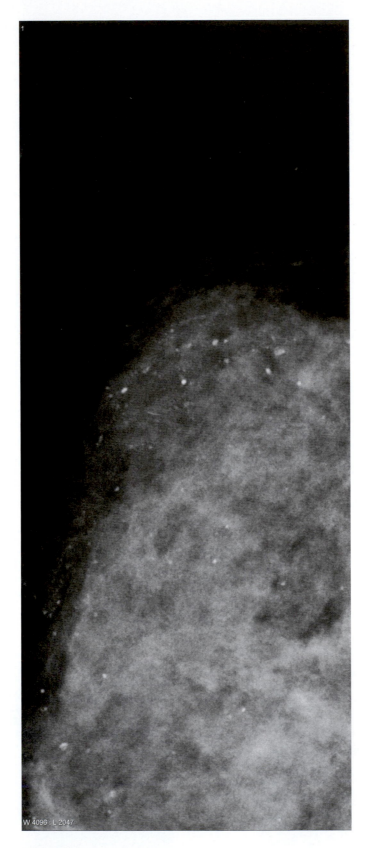

Figure 3–24

ANSWERS AND RATIONALES

1. **(D)**   The skin of the breast is thinnest at the region of the areola, approximately 0.5 mm, and thickest at the base of the breast, approximately 2.0 mm.

2. **(B)**   Breast tissue is located on the anterior chest wall between the 2nd rib and 6/7th rib and from the lateral margin of the sternum to the axilla.

3. **(D)**   Morgagni's tubercles are the surface element of the Montgomery's glands that provide lubrication released during the breast feeding process.

4. **(C)**   The deep fascia separates the pectoralis muscle from the mammary tissue. The deep fascia courses anteriorly from the base of the breast to encase mammary stroma.

5. **(B)**   Cooper's ligaments are a support network of fibrous bands that extend from the base of the breast to the nipple. Eventually over time, this network loses its elastic nature, failing to maintain the shape of the breast.

6. **(B)**   As surrounding breast tissue is invaded by a malignancy, Cooper's ligaments may retract, causing the skin surface to appear dimpled or puckered. Patients who present with a skin surface appearance such as this may have an underlying malignant pathology. Furthermore, with age, Cooper's ligaments naturally lose their elasticity, causing an overall external pendulous appearance.

7. **(B)**   The nipple serves as a point of intersection to divide the breast into 4 quadrants. The majority of actual breast tissue is located in the central and the upper outer quadrant. A 7:00 lesion in the right breast corresponds to the LOQ, whereas a 7:00 lesion in the left breast would correspond to the LIQ.

8. **(C)**   Each lobe of the breast consists of smaller lobulated segments of breast tissue that have a respective duct that courses towards the nipple. The terminal ductal lobular unit is found within the lobules. The intralobular unit is lined with epithelial cells which often become a site for potential pathology. The intralobular terminal unit also houses the acini or ductules.

9. **(D)**   A TDLU consists of both an intralobular terminal unit and an extralobular terminal unit. The intralobular unit is connected to the extralobular terminal unit which anastamose with other surrounding ducts as they course towards the nipple. TDLUs' size and number are influenced by alteration in hormone levels such as with pregnancy, lactation, menopause, and hormone supplements.

10. **(C)**   The lateral thoracic artery and internal mammary artery are branches of the brachiocephalic artery that courses to feed the upper extremities. Therefore, intercostal arteries, the internal mammary artery, and the lateral thoracic artery are all sources of blood supply to the breast.

11. **(B)**   Each breast is divided into four quadrants, using the nipple as the point of intersection. In addition, lesions within the breast can be referenced by a clock system notation. The 5:00 lesion in the left breast corresponds to the LOQ, whereas the 5:00 lesion in the right breast corresponds to the LIQ.

12. **(C)**   Papillomas are a result of overgrowth of epithelial cells found lining the duct. The cells grow in a cluster like fashion off of a stalk. Typically, this pathology is benign in nature, found in the subareolar region, and could potentially cause nipple discharge if it were to grow large enough.

13. **(C)**   Microcalcifications that tend to appear indistinct, irregular in size and shape, and continue to increase in number over a period of time are all indications of a possible malignancy. Pathologies that present with spiculations or stellate borders can also be very strong indicators of a malignancy. Malignancies also have a tendency to present with increased density compared to its surrounding tissue. Macrocalcifications are typically a result of involuting fibroadenomas, therefore signature a benign process.

14. **(C)**   Radial scars may appear mammographically with a stellate border, but with a radiolucent center. If this pathology was noted, it may be necessary for further diagnostic work-up.

15. **(C)**   Inflammatory carcinoma fails to present with a palpable mass. This rapid growing cancer blocks the lymphatic channels of the breast, causing the patient to present with symptoms similar to those of mastitis.

16. **(C)**   Lipomas are benign, fatty tumors that are encapsulated and located superficially around the periphery of the breast.

17. **(A)** DCIS may be noted with ductal calcification found within the duct of a lobe or segment of breast tissue. Calcifications may also be noted within the vessels in which atherosclerosis has taken place.

18. **(B)** There are variety of characteristics that aid in the distinction of probable benign calcifications such as their size, shape, and distribution. Typically, the more dispersed and larger the calcifications are with an egg shelled appearance, the more likely they are benign.

19. **(A)** The milk-producing unit of the breast is within the acini, also known as ductules, found within the lining of the intralobular terminal unit.

20. **(C)** The inframammary fold is where the base of the breast meets the anterior abdominal tissue around the level of the sixth or seventh rib.

21. **(D)** Genetic predisposition may affect the amount of glandular tissue within the breast. In addition, extreme weight gain or loss will alter the ratio of glandular tissue to adipose tissue within the breast. Monthly cyclic changes can cause changes in breast size due to interstitial fluid accumulation.

22. **(D)** Nipple inversion may be associated as part of normal breast development or with development of pathology. Skin that presents with redness may be an indication of infection or an underlying carcinoma such as inflammatory carcinoma. Skin that presents thickened with dimpling results from the retraction of Cooper's ligaments due to a nearby invasion. Nipple discharge may be associated with either benign or malignant disease processes which may warrant further diagnostic work-up.

23. **(B)** Progesterone is the hormone responsible for lobular proliferation and growth. Estrogen is responsible for ductal proliferation. Follicular stimulating hormone (FSH) is a hormone released by the pituitary gland to stimulate ovarian follicles to mature prior to ovulation. Human chorionic gonadotropin (HCG) is a hormone released into the blood stream with the establishment of a placenta site.

24. **(C)** The upper outer quadrant tends to see a higher incidence of breast cancer because of its large volume of tissue and because it is the quadrant which undergoes the slowest regression. Lymphatic channels run throughout the breast and are not associated with UOQ incidence cancers.

25. **(B)** Calcifications noted with increased density or a mass are of concern. Calcifications that are unilateral and grow in a cluster over a period of time are also of concern.

26. **(B)** HRT may be utilized by women suffering from menopausal symptoms. HRT uses estrogen alone or in combination with progesterone to supply the body hormones like the functioning ovaries once did. Therefore, in women of the menopausal age category and older it is possible to see a reappearance of glandular tissue in some areas of the breast.

27. **(B)** As breasts undergo the involution process, breast tissue distribution is compared right to left. Breasts should somewhat mirror one another. An instance where a new density appears unilaterally and this area was not evident on previous mammograms would warrant further investigation with other diagnostic procedures.

28. **(C)** In mammography there is what is referred to as the zero yield factor for certain age category females. Younger females (below 30) tend to have breast tissue that is extremely dense, therefore it is difficult for mammography to achieve adequate separation of tissues, making structure visualization difficult. Therefore, other diagnostic options such as ultrasound should be sought for these patients.

29. **(D)** Lymph nodes can be visible structures within the axillary region. Normal nodes are considered to be oval in shape, 2 cm in length, and have a radiolucent center.

30. **(A)** Morgagni's tubercles are the surface element of the Montgomery's glands that aid in the release of lubrication in the breast feeding process.

31. **(D)** Inflammatory breast cancer can be misdiagnosed as mastitis and the patient could initially receive improper treatment with antibiotics for mastitis. Mastitis and IBC present with similar physical symptoms such as a swollen and inflamed breast without the presence of a palpable lump. IBC is a rapid growing carcinoma with a poor prognosis.

32. **(D)** The film represents a tangential view to determine the location of suspicious calcifications visualized during standard mammography. The outcome of this film would verify dermal or skin calcifications.

33. **(C)** The acinus is represented within the intraductal terminal unit.

34. **(B)**

35. **(C)**

36. **(D)** Microcysts that present with mixture of fluid and calcified particles. Typically are benign unless noted with other associated findings. Milk of calcium is a benign process that can be determined by imaging the patient with a CC and a true 90 degree lateral projection.

4

Mammographic Techniques and Image Evaluation

TECHNICAL FACTORS FOR MAMMOGRAPHY

Technique

There are five basic technical factors involved with mammography. The mammographer will evaluate these for each patient. They are kVp, mAs, density setting, placement of the photocell, and amount of compression. Technical capabilities of machines may vary but the standards are as follows:

1. Different target types will produce different ranges of kVp. It is imperative that the mammography unit allows increases in kVp one increment at a time. Ranges for molybdenum targets are usually 24–30 kVp while rhodium targets have a range of 26–32 kVp. kVp controls the quality of the beam and radiographic contrast.

2. Using the ALARA principle, the mA and time(s) will work together to achieve an optimal mammogram. mAs controls the quantity of electrons hitting the target and is responsible for beam quantity. mAs may be fixed or variable. Machines may have the ability to set mA stations from 20 to 100. However, mAs should always be kept as low as possible. Time should be kept as short as possible to avoid motion and image blur. Remember that reciprocity law failure (RLF)occurs at long exposures and very short exposures. Reciprocity law failure is the failure of density to remain the same over a number of exposures while the exposure factors remain constant. Reciprocity law failure will occur most often with exposure times longer than 1.0 second. Because the silver halide crystals cannot help create a stable image or density on the film, reciprocity law failure may occur. This is due to ability or inability to process the light photon. Different levels of exposure allow for different levels of chemical processing and light absorption. As exposure time increases, the density on the film will not increase linearly.

3. Setting the density control is related to the density of the breast tissue being irradiated. To produce an optimal density, a density regulator is used. Each step will translate into a 0.15 increase or decrease in the OD of the film.

4. Nine density adjustment steps should be available to the mammographer. These include the ability to increase and decrease the density. These adjustments of the photocell correspond to the densest portion of the breast. The photocells must be placed over the densest portions of the breast in order to receive an OD of not less than 1.00 or not greater than 3.00.

5. Breast compression is used to reduce the thickness of the breast thus reducing overall exposure to the patient.

6. Back-up timers are used in mammography and conventional radiography. For nongrid techniques, the back-up times should be set at 300 mAs and 600 mAs for grid techniques. The low energy photons used in mammography have a harder time penetrating the breast, especially with large and dense breast tissues. It is important to note that if the back-up timer is reached you should not increase the density settings; rather the kVp should be increased.

7. Automatic exposure control or AEC can be used in most mammographic situations. However, when imaging patients with breast implants or those patients with very little breast tissue, AEC should not be used. If AEC is used during implant imaging, the back-up timer will be reached and the machine exposure will shut off.

AEC

The goal of AEC is to provide consistent radiation exposure for the range of kVp and for the tissue exposed. Because such a wide range of tissue densities are exposed, there is a great need for AEC. AEC is predetermined. When radiation passes through the object it will be converted to an electrical signal. This signal will reach the detector and terminate the exposure. The AEC detectors can move from the level of the nipple to the chest wall. Most will have 9–10 positions along nipple to chest wall. The ACR uses a phantom to measure the OD produced by the detector. It is mandatory the OD be a minimum of 1.20.

COMPRESSION

As noted before, compressing the patient's breast allows for better visualization of structures, immobilization of the breast, reduced breast thickness, and reduced exposure to the patient. Compression also reduces magnification of structures within the breast by bringing them closer to the image receptor (IR). This includes pathology that may be better visualized through compression (Figure 4–1).

Breast Compression

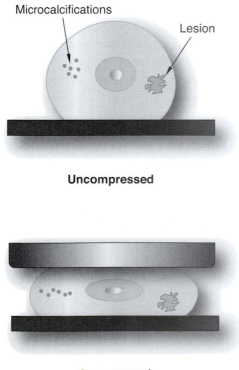

Figure 4–1   Compression

A compression plate is utilized which must allow for uniform compression throughout the breast. It is made of a thin polycarbonate plastic. The compression device should have a straight wall edge, and rest flat and parallel to the image receptor. The height of the compression lip should be at least 2 inches in order to prevent tissue from spilling over onto the breast and projecting into the image. The lip should be placed so as to be perpendicular to the chest wall of the patient. Compression plates also have automatic and hand-controlled abilities to compress. Mammographic units utilize foot pedals to automatically compress the patient's breast and hand-controlled devices to make small incremental compression changes. The compression device should always release once the exposure has been made. MQSA requirements state that compression should not exceed 25–45 lbs or 111–200 newtons.

MAGNIFICATION TECHNIQUE

Magnification technique is employed in mammography to image small areas (Figure 4-2). Because these areas may consist of microcalifications, proper magnification technique is crucial in mammography. Magnification technique does increase patient dose. However, it also allows for the inspection of microcalifications by evaluating their size, number, margins, and dispersion.

The procedure for magnification mammography requires a special magnification attachment. This

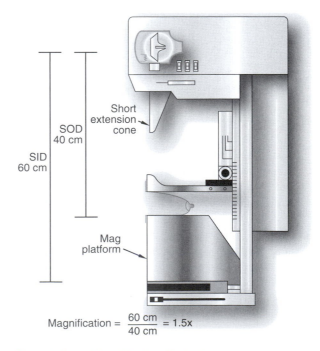

$$\text{Magnification} = \frac{60 \text{ cm}}{40 \text{ cm}} = 1.5x$$

Figure 4–2   Magnification Technique

attaches to the bucky and looks much like a platform. OID is the principle used to magnify the image. It should be noted that magnification technique will increase skin dose while decreasing glandular dose. A small focal spot must be employed to obtain better detail and visualization of structures.

EVALUATION OF THE IMAGE

Evaluation of the image is dependent on many factors including but not limited to positioning, compression, exposure, contrast, sharpness, noise, artifacts, collimation, and image labeling.

When evaluating the image, it is imperative that the *positioning* be evaluated for the specific tissue required for the examination. For instance, in the CC images, the anterior, medial, and central portions of the breast are evaluated while the MLO is an excellent source for posterior and upper outer quadrant tissue evaluation.

- **Compression**, as noted before, is imperative. Proper compression will aid in sharpening the image and structures of the breast as well as reduce patient exposure.

- **Contrast** is best achieved with the proper use of kVp. Differential absorption allows for enhanced contrast. Remember that high contrast images are being employed in mammography with low energy x-ray photons.

- **Sharpness** is the ability to see and enhance fine detail. The number of line pairs per mm of a mammography system should range from 11 to 13. Sharpness is enhanced when slower speed screens are used, OID is kept to a minimum, and SID is maximum.

- **Image noise** is usually caused in mammography from quantum mottle or artifacts. Quantum mottle, the lack of sufficient x-rays to form the image, will also add to noise as will faster film screen combinations. Radiographic mottle may be due to film graininess, which is directly related to the grains of silver halide. Quantum mottle is also determined by film speed and contrast, and absorption abilities of the screen. With faster screens quantum mottle is more obvious. Although, faster screens in any form of radiography decrease dose to the patient.

- **Optimal exposure** requires that all the anatomy be penetrated correctly. OD on the radiograph should be above 1.0.

- **Artifacts** are items or marks on the radiograph that are NOT variants due to the anatomy or pathology but usually due to processing or handling. Some of these include roller marks, finger prints, scratches on the screen, and dirt on the screen. Artifacts not due to the processor, but due to patient factors may include the wearing of perfume powder or deodorant. Hair or body fat in the image receptor (IR) will be visualized. Equipment may also cause artifacts. The most common artifact on a film is grid lines. Other artifacts found in the tube head are misaligned collimator, dust, crooked or uneven mirrors, and faulty compression devices. Artifacts on the tube head will look blurry, as they are far away from the area of interest. Artifacts or marks on the image due to processor handling do not appear blurry. Processor artifacts are usually located by observing the direction of the artifact on the film. Some of the processor marks found are roller marks, guide shoe marks, and chatter.

- **Collimation** is not necessary in mammography. The tube should automatically collimate to the size of the cassette and the mammographer should not further collimate to the breast itself.

- **Labeling** of mammograms is specific to the MQSA rules. The patient name and an additional patient identifier, which may be date of birth or a specific patient ID number, date of the examination, view and laterality, facility name and location, unit the mammogram is performed on, the technologist performing the examination (markers), and cassette/screen identification are required.

REVIEW QUESTIONS

Directions: Choose the word or statement that best completes each question.

1. The normal range of kVp using a molybdenum target is which of the following?

   A. 24–30 kVp

   B. 31–38 kVp

   C. 39–40 kVp

   D. 22–40 kVp

2. In mammography, mAs should be kept as _____ as possible and time should be kept as _____ as possible.

   A. high, short

   B. low, short

   C. low, long

   D. high, long

3. The height of the compression paddle lip should be a minimum of _____.

   A. 1 inch

   B. 2 inches

   C. 3 inches

   D. 4 inches

4. MQSA requires that the compression device have the ability to provide a minimum of _____ lbs/newtons of pressure.

   A. 10/200

   B. 25/111

   C. 44/220

   D. 45/200

5. Compression will increase which of the following?

   1. Sharpness

   2. Visibility of detail

   3. Density

   A. 1 and 2 only

   B. 2 and 3 only

   C. 1 & 3 only

   D. 1, 2, & 3

6. Decreasing kVp will _____ the quality of the beam.

   A. increase

   B. decrease

   C. not change

   D. none of the above

7. Which of the following is not a form of mammographic labeling required by MQSA?

   A. Identification of the technologist flashed on the film

   B. Identification of the angle and projection flashed on the film

   C. Identification of the date flashed on the film

   D. Stickers

8. Which of the following is utilized when compressing the breast?

   1. Motorized compression

   2. Digital compression

   3. Hand-adjusted compression

   A. 1 & 2 only

   B. 1 & 3 only

   C. 1, 2, & 3

   D. All of the above

9. The most common magnification factor utilized in mammography is

   A. 1.0

   B. 1.5

   C. 3.0

   D. 3.5

10. The _____ is a technique used in mammography which reduces the amount of scatter reaching the image receptor.

    A. air gap

    B. platform

    C. scatter

    D. reduction

11. Using a long SID will do what to the sharpness of the image?

    A. Increase

    B. Decrease

    C. There is no change

    D. Decrease by one-third

12. Which type of contrast is preferred in mammography?

    A. High contrast

    B. Low contrast

    C. Low density

    D. High density

13. There are different target/filter combinations which can be used in mammography. Which type of target/filter combination is used for fatty breasts?

    A. Molybdenum/molybdenum

    B. Rhodium/molybdenum

    C. Rhodium/rhodium

    D. Yttrium

14. The ability to see small calcifications and other objects within the breast can be defined as which of the following?

    A. Definition

    B. Image sharpness

    C. Resolution

    D. Clarity

15. To increase contrast on an image (shorter scale), kVp should be

    A. increased

    B. decreased

    C. left the same

    D. doubled

16. Which of the following factors will not add to geometric unsharpness?

    A. Motion

    B. Focal spot

    C. Film blur

    D. Compression

17. _____ occurs when an insufficient number of photons reaches the intensifying screen.

    A. High photon conversion

    B. Chatter

    C. Quantum mottle

    D. Increased contrast

18. Quantum mottle can be overcome by

    A. decreasing kVp

    B. increasing kVp

    C. increasing mAs

    D. decreasing mAs

19. Which of the following factors does not contribute to radiographic noise?

    A. Quantum mottle

    B. Scatter radiation

    C. Size of silver halide crystals

    D. OID (object image distance)

20. Which of the following is the ability to distinguish structures with similar contrast?

    A. Spatial resolution

    B. Sharpness

    C. Contrast resolution

    D. Clarity

21. Which of the following is a major concern in magnification mammography?

    A. Compression

    B. Patient dose

    C. Increased noise

    D. Increased scatter

22. Which of the following is true for implant imaging with the implant displaced?

    A. AEC must be used

    B. Manual technique should be used

    C. Normal positioning is used

    D. Maximum compression is applied

23. Which of the following is not one of the three primary breast tissue types?

    A. Adipose

    B. Fibroglandular

    C. Fibrous

    D. Glandular

24. Which of the following is the most common type of anode material used in mammography?

    A. Molybdenum

    B. Rhodium

    C. Tungsten

    D. Aluminum

25. Which of the following target materials has a kVp range of 26–32 kVp?

    A. Molybdenum

    B. Rhodium

    C. Tungsten

    D. Aluminum

26. Exposure times that exceed _____ second(s) may cause reciprocity law failure.

    A. 0.5

    B. 1.0

    C. 1.5

    D. 2.0

27. Application of _____ requires less kVp, reduces scatter radiation, and reduces breast thickness.

    A. compression

    B. grids

    C. resolution

    D. detail

28. When changing the density increments on the machine, increasing by one increment will change the OD by how much?

    A. 1.0

    B. 0.2

    C. 1.5

    D. 0.15

29. The automatic mode of compression should not exceed _____ of compression force.

    A. 55 lbs

    B. 45 lbs

    C. 35 lbs

    D. 25 lbs

30. For a grid technique, which of the following back-up times should be used?

    A. 100 mAs

    B. 300 mAs

    C. 400 mAs

    D. 600 mAs

ANSWERS AND RATIONALES

1. **(A)**   Most common clinical kVp for a molybdenum target is between 24 and 30 kVp but can vary depending on the unit.

2. **(B)**   mAs should always be kept as low as possible to increase detail, and time should be kept as short as possible to decrease motion.

3. **(B)**   The height of the compression paddle lip should be at least 2 inches in order to prevent tissue from spilling over into the field of interests.

4. **(B)**   MQSA requirements state that a minimum compression of 25 lbs or 111 newtons should be achievable.

5. **(A)**   Compression will increase detail and contrast and decrease density.

6. **(B)**   kVp determines the quality and therefore the penetrating power of the beam. By increasing kVp, a shorter wavelength and greater photon energy is produced. Decreasing kVp would result in more absorption of the photon.

7. **(D)**   Identification highly or strongly suggested by the FDA is by use of the flashcard system. Stickers are not suggested. The following should be included: date, view and laterality, name and other patient identifier, facility name and location (city state and zip code), technologist identification, unit, cassette and screen identification.

8. **(B)**   Compression can be done by utilizing a motorized compression device controlled by a foot peddle and a hand device for small adjustments.

9. **(B)**   The most common magnification factor used in mammography is 1.5 times.

10. **(A)**   The air gap is a technique specifically used to reduce the amount of scatter reaching the IR. A grid is not used with the air gap technique.

11. **(A)**   Increasing SID will reduce magnification therefore improve image sharpness.

12. **(A)**   High contrast film is preferred in mammography as it exhibits greater visibility of detail and greater contrast within structures.

13. **(A)**   For thin fatty type breast tissues, molybdenum is preferred as it creates a photon energy level which will penetrate but not over-penetrate the tissue.

14. **(B)**   Image sharpness is the ability to see small objects/anatomies within the breast.

15. **(B)**   When kVp decreases, the contrast of an image will increase.

16. **(D)**   Compression will actually decrease blurring of the image and tissues.

17. **(C)**   Quantum mottle is an occurrence due to an insufficient number of photons which then do not activate a sufficient number of phosphors. This causes a mottled appearance on the film.

18. **(C)**   Increasing mAs is the only way to decrease quantum mottle.

19. **(D)**   OID will add to image magnification but not to radiographic noise.

20. **(C)**   Spatial resolution is the ability to see differences in structures on a mammogram. Sharpness is detail within the image. Contrast resolution is the ability to distinguish different structures with similar contrast.

21. **(B)**   Increased dose is a concern in magnification mammography, as the radiation exposure to the breast can increase 2–3 times during one single exposure.

22. **(B)**   Manual technique should always be used with implant patients and those patients with very little breast tissue.

23. **(B)**   Fibroglandular is a mixed tissue type and not one of the three main tissue types.

24. **(A)**   Molybdenum is the most common target material used.

25. **(B)**   Rhodium has a kVp range of 26 through 32 kVp.

26. **(B)**   Reciprocity law failure can occur with exposures that exceed 1.0 second.

27. **(A)**   Compression is used to reduce magnification, reduce tissue thickness, reduce exposure, and reduce motion and unsharpness therefore increasing visualization of the image.

28. **(D)**   Each step of density increment on the machine will increase the OD 0.15 times.

29. **(B)**   MQSA guidelines designate that the initial automatic compression mode applied to the breast must be between 111 and 200 newtons or 15–45 pounds, but should not exceed 45 pounds. Too little compression will not result in a good image and too much compression may harm the patient.

30. **(D)**   For a grid technique the back-up timer should be set at 600 mAs. For nongrid techniques, mAs should be set at 300.

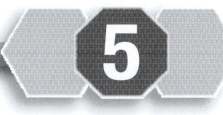

Breast Positioning and Special Procedures

ROUTINE BREAST POSITIONING

The craniocaudal (CC) and mediolateral (MLO) oblique projections are standard complimentary projections utilized for screening mammography. Although, the two projections do not provide a 90 degree view from one another, the MLO allows positioning to include the upper outer quadrant (UOQ) to the inframammary fold (IMF).

Craniocaudal Projection (CC)

The standard CC projection best demonstrates tissue in the subareolar, central, medial, and posterior medial region. This projection poorly demonstrates lateral and posterior lateral breast tissue. On some patients, the pectoralis muscle may in fact be visible on the film. The posterior nipple line (PNL) should measure within 1 cm of the mediolateral oblique projection.

Mediolateral Oblique Projection (MLO)

The MLO projection best demonstrates the posterior and lateral breast tissue along with the upper quadrant of the breast. The IMF should be open and pectoralis muscle should extend to the posterior nipple line. Adequate demonstration of breast tissue will directly reflect positioning. It is imperative that the image receptor be placed parallel to the pectoralis muscle, whether this employs the average 45 degree angle, or more or less dependent on patient body habitus. The pectoralis muscle should appear wider at the level of the axilla and narrow as it courses inferiorly. In addition, good positioning evidences the pectoralis muscle with a convex margin and it extends to

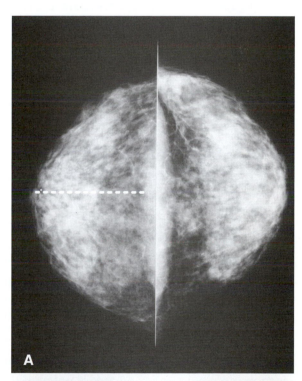

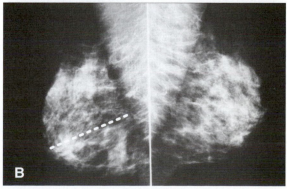

Figure 5–1 (A) Posterior Nipple Line Measurement, (B) Posterior Nipple Line Measurement

the level of the nipple or below. If positioned properly, this single projection alone is ideal to visualize the maximum amount of breast tissue.

To assess breast positioning, a PNL measurement can be acquired on both the CC and MLO and compared (Figure 5–1). CC PNL measurements are acquired by measuring perpendicularly from the nipple to either the edge of the film or the anterior edge of the pectoralis muscle. MLO PNL measurements are acquired by measuring perpendicularly from the nipple to the anterior edge of the pectoralis muscle. PNL measurements that correspond within 1 cm between the CC and MLO aid in the determination that adequate breast tissue has been imaged.

ADDITIONAL BREAST IMAGING

There are a variety of additional projections that may be acquired to better demonstrate tissues or areas of interest in the breast. In addition, special imaging projections may be helpful to better demonstrate a suspicious area within the breast or when a lesion may only be seen on one view. Furthermore, additional breast imaging may help avoid an invasive procedure for a patient. Lesions within the breast may be localized with an additional projection such as a 90 degree lateral along with the standard projections to determine their location.

Mediolateral (ML) and the Lateromedial (LM) Projection

The ML or LM projections are orthogonal views (90 degrees) to the CC. The projection implemented depends on the area within the breast that is of primary interest. The area of interest needs to be placed closest to the image receptor to maximize resolution of the structures. In other words, a LM projection is of choice when an area is noted in the more medial aspect of the breast. A true lateral projection also assists with localization of lesions by noting their position in relation to the nipple. Lesions that move more superiorly in the breast in reference to the nipple on the lateral will indicate a more medial lesion. Lesions that move more inferiorly in the breast in reference to the nipple on the lateral indicate a more lateral lesion. Lesions that do not change position significantly from a MLO projection to a 90 degree lateral would indicate a more centrally located lesion. True 90 degree projections serve useful to reference structures in relationship to the nipple. However, these projections are a poor

means to demonstrate the posterior and lateral tissue areas of the breast.

Triangulation Technique

In instances in which two projections demonstrate an abnormality, a triangulation technique can be applied to determine an approximate location. A lesion visualized in two projections can be triangulated by measuring straight back from the nipple to intersect with the lesion, on each projection. These two lines will intersect the approximate area of the lesion allowing a quadrant and a clock time to be determined. In instances in which only one projection demonstrates an abnormality, the triangulation technique is not applicable.

Exaggerated Craniocaudal (XCCL)

This additional projection is somewhat similar to a standard CC projection, but rather than focusing on the medial aspect of the breast, patient positioning is modified to image tissue within the posterior and lateral edge of the breast. Undoubtedly, deep medial breast tissue will be compromised as the patient's posterior and lateral tissue regions are pulled into view. In certain instances, a slight tube angle, approximately 5 degrees in the MLO direction, is helpful to avoid interference with the humeral head. The central ray is directed midway between the nipple and the lateral edge of the breast.

Spot Compression

Spot compression imaging is helpful in imaging a suspicious finding located within a dense tissue region. Spot compression projections will require the standard compression paddle to be replaced with a smaller compression device. The smaller compression device results in increased focal compression to a marked area of suspicion to improve resolution (Figure 5–2).

Spot compression will be applied according to the lesion's location. By viewing either the CC or the MLO, the lesion may be localized by first measuring directly posterior to the nipple to stop at the level of the lesion. From the stopping point of the first lesion, acquire a second measurement either superior or inferior (MLO) or medial or lateral (CC) position to the lesion. A CC aids in localizing lesions in either medial or lateral positions in the breast while the MLO aids

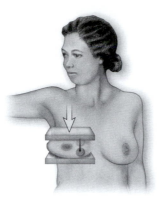

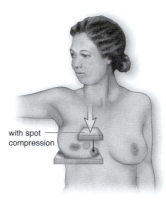

with spot compression

Figure 5–2   Spot Compression

in localizing lesions superior and inferior to the nipple. Lastly, a measurement from the lesion to the skin margin should be acquired. The acquired measurements can then be applied to the breast and marked to aid supplemental imaging.

Magnification Imaging

Magnification projections are acquired to better determine the margins of lesions or to better evaluate calcifications. A magnification tower will be secured to the unit and localization and spot compression may or may not be used. Magnification imaging does not require the use of a grid, as the air-gap technique is implemented.

Caudocranial or Reverse CC or From Below (FB)

The caudocranial projection serves as a useful substitution for the standard CC or a supplemental view to the CC if necessary. The reverse CC may be useful when working with male patients, kyphotic patients, localizing a lesion located inferiorly within the breast, or for better visualization of a superiorly located lesion. The positioning for this projection is the same as the standard CC, except that the C-arm is rotated 180 degrees and special attention should be directed to the abdominal tissue to avoid superimposition.

Axillary Tail (AT)

This additional projection is employed when a special look at the axillary tail or the Tail of Spence is warranted. The C-Arm is rotated with a 10–30 degree angle to become parallel with the axillary tail. The patient is positioned similarly to the MLO, but this projection

can not replace the MLO projection. The central ray should be between the nipple and axilla.

Cleavage (CV)

This projection requires the positioning of both breasts on the image receptor with or without compression. The projection best visualizes deep posterior and medial lesions closest to the chest wall. AEC may be implemented with adequate tissue positioned over the photocell. Breasts may be positioned with the cleavage off-center to allow for tissue coverage according to the photocell. In instances where this may not be the case, manual technical factors should be set for the exposure (Figure 5–3).

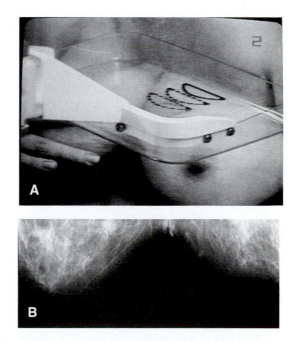

Figure 5–3   (A) Cleavage Positioning, (B) Cleavage Projection

Rolled Views

Rolled lateral (RL) or rolled medial (RM) views are utilized when breast tissue superimposes a lesion or area of interest. RL projections roll the superior region of the breast laterally and the inferior region medially from a standard CC position. RM projections roll the superior breast region medially and the inferior region laterally from a standard CC position. Again, the RL and RM views are helpful to move dense breast tissue from an area of a suspicious lesion or may be implemented to truly determine if there is in fact a lesion present. If a density is still noted after the roll, then the area seen on the mammogram is real.

Rolled views can assist with lesion localization. On a craniocaudal rolled medial (CCRM), a density that positions itself in the medial half of the breast reveals the lesion is located in the superior breast, as that was the direction the superior tissue was rolled. On the other hand, if a CCRM projection positions the lesion in the lateral breast, the lesion is located in the inferior tissue, again represented by the direction of the roll.

Rolled views may also be obtained with the breast in a lateral position and then rolled either superiorly (RS) or inferiorly (RI). RS projections require the breast to be truly lateral and then with a counterclockwise rotation of the breast tissue while the RI projections require a clockwise rotation of the tissue (Figure 5–4).

Tangential Projection (TAN)

Tangential projections position the area of interest in such a way that the beam skims across the surface. The beam should be positioned parallel with the structure of interest. Often, this projection is useful in differentiating calcifications within the skin margin (dermal calcifications) or within actual breast tissue located towards the outer margin of the breast. Tangential views may also prove useful in instances in which a palpable lesion (i.e., lump) is within deep glandular tissue. A lead marker (BB) should be placed over the lump and then the beam tangential to the lead marker. In instances of imaging calcifications, the breast is localized with an alphanumeric fenestrated paddle to aid in placement of the lead marker over the calcifications. Once the lead marker is placed, again the x-ray beam is rotated and aligned tangential to the BB.

Lateromedial Oblique (LMO)

This projection may be implemented in instances in which the patient's body habitus poses difficulty for the MLO projection to be acquired. These instances may be patients with pacemakers, pectus excavatum, port-a-caths, defibulators, or patients with recent surgery to the chest cavity. The LMO is a true reverse oblique to the MLO, as the image receptor is placed along the medial aspect of the breast instead of the lateral aspect of the breast. This projection is successful in imaging medial breast lesions with improved resolution.

Superolateral to Inferomedial Oblique (SIO)

The SIO projection requires C-arm angulation of 45 degrees allowing the visualization of the upper inner and lower outer quadrant. The beam is directed from a superior lateral approach towards the inferior and medial breast.

Implant Displaced (ID Views)

Implants may be placed behind or in front of the pectoralis major muscle. Placement of the implant may alter the amount of breast tissue to work with. Regardless, implant patients must be positioned to maximize the amount of breast tissue. Standard CC and MLO views are required both with the implant in place and with the implant displaced. Projections taken with the implant in place will undergo standard positioning requirements, with application of mild compression and the selection of manual technical factors. Implant displaced projections require the actual breast tissue to be manipulated away from the implant and positioned accordingly again with the standard CC and MLO. With the tissue displaced from the implant, adequate compression can be applied to the tissue and exposure may be made with AEC or manual technique if the amount of breast tissue won't adequately cover the AEC detector (Figure 5–5).

PATIENT CIRCUMSTANCES REQUIRING IMAGING MODIFICATION

Patient instances such as body habitus, post surgical conditions, treatment regimens, and chest wall deformities may require special positioning modifications to image the breast without compromising tissue.

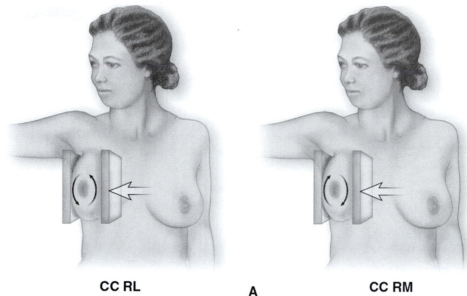

CC RL   A   CC RM

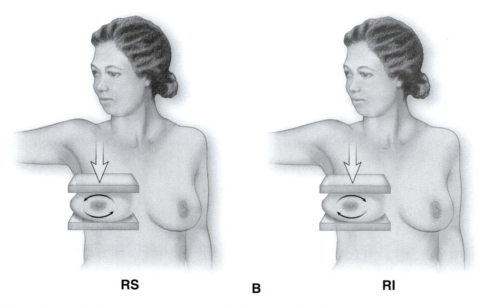

RS   B   RI

Figure 5–4   (A) Rolled Lateral and Medial Positions, (B) Rolled Superior and Inferior Projections

Barrel Chested Patients (Pigeon Breast)

These patients have a protruding chest wall, causing the breast tissue to locate more laterally on the chest wall and even extend underneath the arm. In these instances, it may be difficult to image the breast entirely with the two standard projections. The following is suggested:

- CC performed to assess medial breast tissue.
- XCCL performed to assess extreme lateral breast tissue.
- MLO performed to assess the posterolateral tissue and tissue in the UOQ.

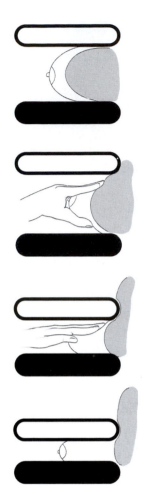

Figure 5–5   Implant Displaced Views

Pectus Excavatum (Sunken Chest)

These patients have hollowing in of the rib cage; the sternum and rib cage tend to be sunken in. This patient will pose an imaging challenge as the entire breast will not likely be assessed through standard imaging procedures. In these instances the medial breast tissue will be difficult to image, therefore, the following is suggested:

■ CC performed for the more medial breast tissue and again for the lateral breast tissue; a CV is also an alternative to image deep medial tissue.

■ LMO likely performed over the MLO for the posterolateral tissue.

■ LM performed to aid in assessment of medial tissue.

Kyphoscoliosis

These patients are characterized with extreme non-symmetric malformations to the vertebral column and rib cage. In these instances, the following is suggested:

■ CC performed with the patient in a seated position to help lengthen the upper body. A CC for the medial tissue may be acquired and then a XCCL performed for the posterior, lateral tissue.

■ MLO or LMO performed for the lateral breast tissue.

■ LM performed for the more extreme posterolateral and posteromedial tissue.

Male Patients

Male patients may present with a body type that would allow the mammography exam to resemble the standard positioning acquired with female patients. However, in instances where males present with small, firm, or very muscular breasts, exam modification is sought. It may be necessary to reduce the amount of compression applied. The following imaging sequence is suggested:

■ Reverse CC or FB projection performed to image medial and lateral aspects of the breast. Be cautious to ensure that abdominal tissue is pulled down and does not superimpose upon the breast tissue.

■ MLO performed for the posterolateral breast tissue.

Surgical or Post-surgical Patients
Post-mastectomy Patients

Post mastectomy patients are strongly encouraged to undergo routine mammography, as local recurrence to the chest wall, lateral chest wall, and axilla may be possible, although imaging this affected side is controversial. Imaging the altered breast side may include a CC, MLO, spot compression, or imaging within the axillary region. Handling the patient carefully physically and emotionally is necessary to minimize patient discomfort (Figure 5–6).

Lumpectomy Patients

Again, imaging lumpectomy patients for recurrence or new potential occurrence with mammography is still advised although rate of recurrence on patients with breast conservation therapy is low. Imaging the

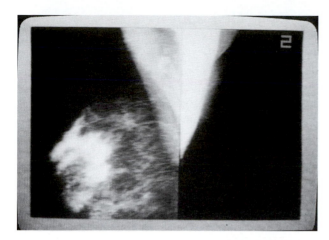

Figure 5–6   Postmastectomy Imaging

altered breast with CC, MLO, or true laterals are all possible. Projections may in fact include magnification views for further evaluation.

Reduction Mammoplasty

A reduction in breast tissue and size is the desired outcome with reduction mammoplasty. The result of this procedure will alter the symmetry of breast tissue comparatively. Women undergoing this procedure undergo mammography prior to the surgery to ensure nothing of concern is noted. Post-surgical procedures to the breast may involve a variety of changes within the breast, including hematomas, calcifications, and fibrous changes.

Pacemakers and Port-a-Caths

Patients with a prominent pacemaker or placement of a port-a-cath will still undergo the standard imaging, but with slight modifications if necessary. A LMO may be substituted for the MLO to avoid the compression paddle along the chest wall.

Irradiated Breast

In some instances, surgical intervention alone may not be in the patient's best interest. There are instances in which adjuvant therapy becomes part of a treatment plan, whether this adjuvant therapy is chemotherapy, radiation therapy, or tamoxifen. Adjuvant therapy is determined by characteristics of the lesion and node involvement. Radiation therapy is commonly administered to patients undergoing breast conservatory therapy to reduce the chance of local recurrence in the nearby tissues. Patients undergoing radiation therapy with orders for a follow-up mammogram will require special handling of the breast. The breast may appear inflamed, swollen, and red.

INTERVENTIONAL PROCEDURES

A variety of interventional procedures may be sought for a patient to aid in achieving a more definitive diagnosis. The selected procedure will depend upon the patient situation and preliminary results.

Needle Localization

The purpose of a needle localization procedure is to preoperatively determine the location of a lesion. Therefore, accurate needle placement is essential, as it guides the surgeon. Needle localization requires needle-wire sets along with a small open or fenestrated compression paddle designed with a grid system to localize a lesion (Figure 5–7). The procedure begins with a scout film acquired with the alphanumeric compression paddle to localize the suspicious area. The radiologist will prep the skin and attempt proper needle placement. Following initial needle placement, another film is acquired to check proper placement. A film is taken each time the needle is repositioned to verify its placement. Once proper placement is achieved, a second projection 90 degrees from the first is acquired. Post verification of the needle placement, a methylene blue dye may be introduced to mark the lesion. Finally, the wire is placed and the needle is removed. The wire is secured and final mammograms are sent with the patient to surgery.

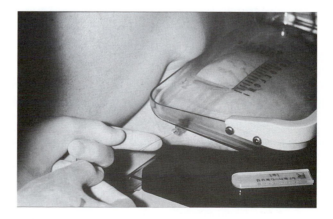

Figure 5–7   Needle Localization

Specimen Radiography

Specimen radiography takes place after a biopsy has been acquired or an excisional biopsy to ensure the lesion and its margins were removed. Specimen filming requires magnification imaging with a factor of 1.5 to 2 times and collimated down to specimen size.

Fine Needle Aspiration Cytology (FNAC)

FNAC is a procedure that may be used to verify malignancy with a suspicious lesion or to confirm a benign lesion. Utilizing FNAC procedure on a benign appearing lesion may avoid the need for a surgical biopsy or could indicate the need for a surgical biopsy. The FNAC procedure is performed under diagnostic guidance, commonly ultrasound or mammography. Regardless of the diagnostic tool utilized, a needle is placed into the lesion and then cellular material is withdrawn into the lumen of the needle. The needle will carefully be removed from the breast and the cellular material is expressed from the needle lumen onto a cytology slide for analysis.

Core Biopsy

A core biopsy procedure will require a larger core of tissue to be removed from the breast. The procedure utilizes an 11–14 gauge needle placed into a rapid firing biopsy gun. Once the needle is placed within the lesion, the biopsy gun is activated to obtain a core sample of tissue. Newer vacuum assisted devices are designed with a rotating cutter and suction to acquire the tissue sample.

Pneumocystography

This procedure initially begins as a standard cyst aspiration with utilization of ultrasound guidance. A needle with an attached syringe is positioned into the lesion. Fluid is first withdrawn from the cyst. Before removal of the needle, the syringe containing cystic fluid is detached from the needle and then a syringe with an equal amount of air is attached and injected into the cyst. Following removal of the needle, CC and ML projections are acquired. This procedure is useful in evaluating the characteristics of a cyst wall that may not have been clearly visible with ultrasound (Figure 5–8).

Ductography

This procedure may also be referred to as galactography and is performed to image the ductal system in instances where patients are experiencing nipple discharge. Nipple discharge that is noted unilaterally and is either bloody or watery is suspicious. The procedure requires the duct secreting the discharge to be isolated and then cannulated. Once the duct is cannulated, contrast material is injected (approximately 1 cc) and the cannula is secured to the chest wall. The patient will then undergo a CC projection with light compression followed by a ML or LM projection if the duct is adequately filling with contrast. Once films are acquired, the cannula is removed and a wet dressing is applied to the breast. The wet dressing aids in draining the contrast from the ductal system to prevent obstruction (Figure 5–9).

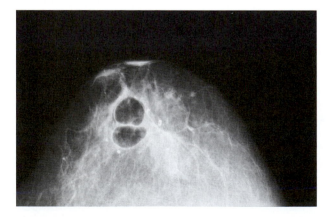

Figure 5–8   Pneumocystography

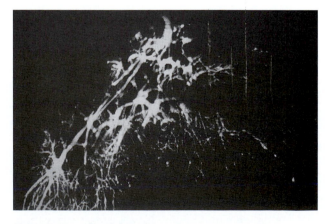

Figure 5–9   Ductography

REVIEW QUESTIONS

Directions: Choose the word or statement that best completes each question.

1. A procedure which aspirates cellular material from a lesion within the breast to undergo a cytology review describes:

    A. core biopsy

    B. cyst aspiration

    C. needle localization

    D. fine needle aspiration

2. A lesion in the lower outer quadrant of the left breast is located at

    A. 2:00 position

    B. 5:00 position

    C. 7:00 position

    D. 9:00 position

3. The most fixed portions of the breast are considered to be

    1. lateral

    2. medial

    3. inferior

    4. superior

    A. 1 and 2

    B. 2 and 3

    C. 1 and 3

    D. 2 and 4

4. Lesions located either medially or laterally to the nipple would be best imaged with a

    A. CC projection

    B. XCCL projection

    C. ML projection

    D. MLO projection

5. The C-arm rotation that may be necessary on a MLO projection with a short, stocky patient is closer to

    A. 15 degrees

    B. 30 degrees

    C. 45 degrees

    D. 60 degrees

6. Which of the following projections would be utilized to best demonstrate a deep medial lesion closely related to the chest wall?

    A. CC

    B. CV

    C. AX

    D. MLO

7. A patient with a prominent pacemaker could be better imaged with

    A. CC and MLO

    B. CC and AX

    C. CC and LMO

    D. CC and XCCL

8. A 6:00 breast lesion may be better demonstrated with which projection?

    A. CC

    B. MLO

    C. AX

    D. ML

9. The ML projection is not considered to be a standard imaging projection because

    A. it is useful to image the 12:00 and 6:00 clock face positions only

    B. it is useful to demonstrate milk of calcium

    C. it fails to demonstrate the posterior and UOQ of the breast

    D. it fails to demonstrate the tissue posterior to the nipple adequately

10. The FB projection may be used when imaging

    1. a patient with reduction mammoplasty

    2. a small breasted male patient

    3. a kyphotic patient

    A. 1 and 2

    B. 2 and 3

    C. 1 and 3

    D. all of the above

11. A PNL measurement that results in a 2 cm difference between the CC and the MLO indicates

    A. adequate positioning and tissue demonstration

    B. improper positioning with failure to demonstrate all the breast tissue

    C. improper positioning, but still displays a majority of the breast tissue

    D. satisfactory imaging, supplemental imaging could be sought

12. A supplemental projection that applies focal compression to the breast to aid in increasing resolution describes

    A. spot compression

    B. TAN compression

    C. ID

    D. CV

13. Suspicious microcalcifications noted in the outer most zone of the breast may require which of the following projections to determine the origination of the microcalcifications?

    A. XCCL

    B. AX

    C. Spot compression

    D. TAN

14. Which of the following would be best to truly determine the margins of a lesion?

    A. Spot compression

    B. TAN

    C. Ultrasound

    D. Magnification

15. Preoperative localization serves to achieve the following:

    1. confirms complete removal of tissue

    2. localizes region for exploratory surgery

    3. localizes the region of tissue to allow for the smallest excision

    A. 1 only

    B. 2 only

    C. 3 only

    D. all of the above

16. Ductal wall abnormalities and growths could be diagnosed with

    A. standard mammography

    B. pneumocystography

    C. FNAC

    D. ductography

17. Ultrasound could be used as

    1. a primary screening tool in patients over 40

    2. a secondary diagnostic tool

    3. a useful means in determining lesions to be cystic or solid

    A. 1 and 2

    B. 1 and 3

    C. 2 and 3

    D. all of the above

18. Pneumocystography proves useful in

    A. demonstrating the true size of the cyst

    B. demonstrating wall characteristics of cysts

    C. determining the true location of the cyst

    D. guiding fluid aspiration

19. Which of the following projections would best image the medial aspect of the breast?

    A. AX

    B. XCCL

    C. MLO

    D. LMO

20. Which of the following supports the need for rolled projections?

    1. In instances when breast tissue of interest is superimposed

    2. In instances when determining something suspicious to be truly something

    3. In instances when not all the breast tissue is included on the film

    A. 1 and 2

    B. 2 and 3

    C. 1 and 3

    D. All of the above

21. The projection utilized to image the tail of the breast is

    A. CC

    B. MLO

    C. XCCL

    D. AT

22. A lesion located more medially in the breast would be best imaged with a _____ 90 degree lateral projection.

    A. ML

    B. LM

    C. AT

    D. XCCL

23. Which of the following supports the reasoning for reestablishing a baseline mammogram prior to the start of radiation therapy for a patient who has undergone BCT?

    A. Breast tissue will be altered from the effects of radiation therapy

    B. Breast tissue will be structurally different following BCT when compared to pre-BCT films

    C. There is no need to reestablish baseline films

    D. The BCT breast will be more difficult to image due to radiation effects

24. Pectus excavatum describes a condition that

    A. causes the patient's chest wall to protrude

    B. causes the patient's chest wall to develop curvature

    C. causes the sternum and medial part of the rib cage to sink inward

    D. none of the above

25. Which portion of the breast would be most difficult to include on a standard CC projection on a patient who is barrel chested?

    A. Medial tissue

    B. Lateral tissue

    C. Superior tissue

    D. Inferior tissue

26. Which of the following projections would be useful in demonstrating lesions located laterally in the breast?

    1. CC
    2. XCCL
    3. ML

    A. 1 and 2

    B. 1 and 3

    C. 2 and 3

    D. All of the above

27. A medial lesion located on the CC and MLO would be expected to move _____ on a 90 degree lateral.

    A. superiorly

    B. inferiorly

    C. laterally

    D. medially

28. In order to position for a MLO projection, the image receptor must be placed parallel with which of the following structures?

    A. Sternum

    B. Axillary tail

    C. Inframammary fold

    D. Pectoralis muscle

29. When positioning a right CC, which arm should reach up to the bar on the C-arm?

    A. Ipsilateral arm

    B. Contralateral arm

    C. Neither arm

    D. Both arms

30. Which portion of the breast is not well visualized on a CC projection?

    A. Central

    B. Medial

    C. Lateral

    D. Posterior medial

31. Which portion of the breast is not well visualized with a MLO projection?

    A. Medial

    B. UOQ

    C. Posterior

    D. All of the above

32. A resultant MLO image demonstrates the pectoralis muscle to be vertical instead of a convex shape. Which of the following would cause this result?

    A. Bucky height too high

    B. Poor muscle relaxation

    C. Incorrect tube angle

    D. Any of the above

33. Screening mammography requires which of the following projections?

    A. CC and ML

    B. CC and XCCL

    C. CC and MLO

    D. CC, MLO, and AT

34. A patient of thin and tall stature would require which of the following angles for a MLO projection?

    A. 30 degrees

    B. 45 degrees

    C. 60 degrees

    D. 80 degrees

35. Which of the following structures must be included on a MLO to ensure the entire breast has been adequately imaged?
    A. Upper Outer Quadrant (UOQ)
    B. Pectoralis muscle
    C. Nipple in profile
    D. Inframammary Fold (IMF)

36. Which one projection of the breast has the likelihood of including the majority of the breast?
    A. CC
    B. ML
    C. MLO
    D. CV

37. Suspicious lesions at either 12:00 or 6:00 would best be demonstrated
    A. with a CC projection
    B. with a MLO projection
    C. with a ML projection
    D. with a CV projection

38. Spot compression provides
    A. focal compression, increasing resolution
    B. diffuse compression, increasing resolution
    C. focal compression, decreasing resolution
    D. diffuse compression, decreasing resolution

39. Which of the following are correct when positioning a XCCL?
    1. Extreme posterolateral tissue pulled into view
    2. Patient positioned in a steep oblique
    3. A slight lateral tube angle applied
    A. 1 and 2
    B. 2 and 3
    C. 1 and 3
    D. All of the above

40. Which of the following should be utilized to best evaluate the characteristics of microcalcifications?
    A. Spot compression views
    B. Rolled views
    C. Magnification views
    D. Tangential views

41. A condition in which the patient's rib cage and sternum are sunken is referred to as
    A. pigeon breast
    B. pectus excavatum
    C. barrel chest
    D. none of the above

42. In which of the following should a baseline film be reestablished?
    A. 49 year old female
    B. 46 year old woman after a FNA
    C. 52 year old woman after a quadrantectomy
    D. 56 year old woman after a stereotactic procedure

43. The central ray for a XCCL film should be
    A. centered to the breast, behind the nipple
    B. centered midway between the nipple and the medial breast margin
    C. centered midway between the nipple and the lateral breast margin
    D. centered midway between the nipple and the inferior breast margin

44. Which of the following projections would better visualize a superior breast lesion?
    A. Caudocranial
    B. Craniocaudal
    C. MLO
    D. SIO

45. The central ray for an AT film should be
    A. centered to the breast, posterior to the nipple
    B. centered between the nipple and the IMF
    C. centered between the nipple and axilla
    D. centered between the medial and lateral breast margins

ANSWERS AND RATIONALES

1. **(D)** FNAC acquires a small sample of cellular material from a lesion to aid in determination of a benign or malignant growth.

2. **(B)** The left lower outer quadrant would include clock face lesions at the 4:00 and 5:00 positions.

3. **(D)** The most immobile portions of the breast are the superior and medial borders while the most mobile portions of the breast are the inferior and lateral borders.

4. **(A)** The CC projection best demonstrates lesions located laterally and medially and extreme medial tissue in relationship to the nipple.

5. **(B)** Patients with a shorter and stockier stature may require a tube angle or rotation such as 30 degrees, which is less than the average patient angle degree. Tall and thin patients may in fact need a C-arm rotation closer to 60 degrees to place the imaging receptor parallel to the pectoralis muscle.

6. **(B)** The cleavage projection (CV) positions both breasts upon the image receptor, allowing the patient to pull herself into the unit. Moderate compression can be applied. Deep medial and posterior lesions are better demonstrated.

7. **(C)** The standard CC can be acquired, but instead of the MLO an LMO could be substituted to avoid the compression paddle making direct contact with the pacemaker.

8. **(D)** A true 90 degree ML or LM will best demonstrate the 12:00 and 6:00 points within the breast.

9. **(C)** The ML is useful to: evaluate 12:00 and 6:00 clock face positions, aid in determination of Milk of Calcium, and demonstrate the location of lesions in relationship to the nipple. However, the ML does a poor job of imaging extreme posterior tissue and tissue that extends from the UOQ into the axilla.

10. **(B)** Small breasted males and kyphotic patients may be successfully imaged with the reverse CC or FB projection.

11. **(B)** PNL measurements between the CC and MLO should correspond within 1 cm, which ensures that a maximum amount of breast tissue has been imaged. When a measurement over 1 cm is evident, projections should be carefully analyzed and a projection selected for a repeat film.

12. **(A)** Spot compression applies compression to a focal area in the breast in efforts to improve the detail of the tissue of question.

13. **(D)** The TAN projection will be useful when determining if microcalcification(s) originate within the skin line of the patient or are in the actual breast parenchyma.

14. **(D)** Magnification imaging is useful to better interpret the margins of a lesion or the characteristics of calcifications.

15. **(C)** Preoperative localization serves to guide the surgeon to the area of suspicion, aiding in the smallest tissue excision as possible. Preoperative localization fails to confirm accurate tissue excision, as this is left to specimen imaging.

16. **(D)** Ductography or galactography will aid in determining the cause of nipple discharge. Nipple discharge that is unilateral may be related to ductal wall abnormalities or growths such as papillomas.

17. **(C)** Ultrasound is a useful diagnostic tool in instances where a palpable mass needs to be differentiated as cystic or solid following a mammography exam. Ultrasound is not advocated as a primary screening means in women over 40. However, ultrasound may be a tool implemented in younger patients suffering from fibrocystic condition or other benign breast lesions that could not be yielded from mammography.

18. **(B)** Pneumocystography is a diagnostic tool that is useful when it comes to evaluation of wall structure of the lesion if ultrasound is incapable of doing so. The procedure includes aspiration of the cyst followed by an injection of air to distend the cavity again for mammography projections.

19. **(D)** Although the MLO and LMO are similar projections, in the instance of this question, the best answer would be the LMO. The LMO positions the medial portion of the breast tissue closest to the image receptor, therefore, improving resolution.

20. **(A)** Rolled medial (RM), rolled lateral (RL), rolled superior (RS), and rolled inferior (RI) may be necessary to better image segments of the breast that are of suspicion and contain tissue superimposition and in instances to determine if a lesion is actually present.

21. **(D)** The AT projection aligns the C-arm with a slight rotation until it is parallel with the AT and centered accordingly to the tail of the breast.

22. **(B)**   A medial lesion will be placed closer to the image receptor with a LM projection, enhancing the resolution of the structure.

23. **(B)**   Reestablishing a baseline for a patient who has undergone breast conservation therapy prior to the start of radiation therapy is useful as the breast tissue may have been structurally altered.

24. **(C)**   Pectus excavatum describes a patient's chest wall to as deformed with an inward depression of the sternum and medial rib cage. Patients with barrel chest are just the opposite and appear with a protrusion of the chest wall.

25. **(B)**   Patients with an extreme barrel chest will have breast tissue that extends out laterally underneath the arm. This type of body habitus will unlikely permit you to image the breast with the standard 2 views. A CC can be acquired for the medial tissue on the chest wall and a XCCL may be needed to include the lateral edge of the breast.

26. **(C)**   Lesions located in the more lateral aspect of the breast would be best imaged utilizing additional views such as the XCCL, ML, and AT in addition to the standard projections.

27. **(A)**   A true medial lesion would be expected to move up or be more superior in the breast on a true 90 degree lateral film. A true lateral lesion would be expected to move down or be inferior on a 90 degree film.

28. **(D)**   The pectoralis muscle should be positioned parallel to the image receptor to ensure adequate positioning of the breast.

29. **(B)**   It is recommended that the contralateral arm to the side being imaged be raised to be secured to the handle in order to help position maximum medial breast tissue.

30. **(C)**   The CC best visualizes central, subareolar, medial, and posteromedial breast tissue.

31. **(A)**   The MLO projection best visualizes the posterior and upper outer quadrant of the breast to compliment the tissue obtained on the CC projection.

32. **(D)**   If the bucky height is too high, this will affect the arm level and the position of the patient, making the pectoralis muscle vertical and making it difficult to pull the breast tissue in. In addition, incorrect tube angle to the patient's body habitus or poor muscle relaxation could result in a film in which the pectoralis muscle is vertical instead of convex.

33. **(C)**   Screening mammography employs the standard CC and MLO projections of each breast. Additional views may be used to supplement if necessary.

34. **(C)**   The tube angle on a MLO projection may vary from patient to patient dependent on body habitus. The tube angle could range between 30 and 60 degrees. An approximate 30 degree tube angle is often used for shorter and wider stature patients, 45–50 degrees is for the average patient, and closer to 60 degrees for the taller and/or thinner patient.

35. **(D)**   The most inferior portion of the breast is noted as being included on the film when the IMF is included on the film.

36. **(C)**   The MLO is the best projection to get the majority of the breast on one film, as the UOQ, IMF, and posterior breast are visualized.

37. **(C)**   12:00 or 6:00 suspicious lesions would be best visualized with a true lateral projection (LM or ML).

38. **(A)**   Focal compression will increase the image resolution where compression is applied. Spot compression is useful in evaluating areas of suspicion.

39. **(C)**   When positioning a XCCL, the tissue of interest is posterior and lateral. This tissue should be pulled into view by slightly obliquing the breast, and a slight 5 degree lateral tube angle may be applied to avoid the humeral head in the projection.

40. **(C)**   Magnification views are applied to imaging margins of a lesion or characteristics of calcifications.

41. **(B)**   Pectus excavatum describes a sunken rib cage and sternum making standard positioning difficult. Patients referred to as barrel or pigeon breasted have a protruding chest wall, again making standard positioning a challenge.

42. **(C)**   Alteration to the breast tissue such as with a lumpectomy or quadrantectomy with or without follow-up radiation therapy require reestablishing a baseline film.

43. **(C)**   XCCL positioning will better visualize the posteromedial breast, therefore centering midway between the nipple and the lateral margin of the breast is appropriate.

44. **(A)**   The caudocranial or FB projection would allow the superior portion of the breast to be positioned closer to the image receptor, improving the resolution of the structure.

45. **(C)**   The AT view will best visualize the axillary tail of the breast. It will require centering to fall midway between the level of the nipple and the axilla.

6

Practice Examination

1. The inferior part of the breast on a MLO may not attain proper compression when
   A. the patient is inadequately turned into the machine
   B. too much of the patient's shoulder and axilla is compressed
   C. improper tube angulation is used
   D. the patient's breast is too large

2. In the automatic mode of compression application, the unit should be able to obtain
   A. between 20 and 24 lbs
   B. between 25 and 45 lbs
   C. between 30 and 50 lbs
   D. between 40 and 45 lbs

3. A sentinel node is described as
   A. a node containing cancer
   B. a node with no trace of metastasis
   C. the first node that receives drainage from the tumor
   D. the last node that receives drainage from the tumor

4. Cyclic hormone(s) that prepare the breasts for possible pregnancy each month is/are
   1. estrogen
   2. testosterone
   3. progesterone
   A. 1 only
   B. 1 and 2
   C. 2 and 3
   D. 1 and 3

5. The atrophy of breast tissue first begins
   A. superiorly and laterally
   B. anteriorly and laterally
   C. posteriorly and medially
   D. posterior to the nipple

6. A screen film contact QC test that displays multiple small areas (less than 1 cm in diameter) of poor contact would require which of the following actions?
   A. replace the screens in the cassette
   B. remove the cassette from clinical use
   C. return the cassette into clinical use
   D. re-clean the screens and repeat the test

7. Increased kVp will produce which of the following effects?
   A. High contrast
   B. Low contrast
   C. Increased patient dose
   D. Increased resolution

8. The projection that is most useful to demonstrate the superior or inferior relationship of structures to the nipple is
   A. TAN
   B. ML
   C. CC
   D. rolled views

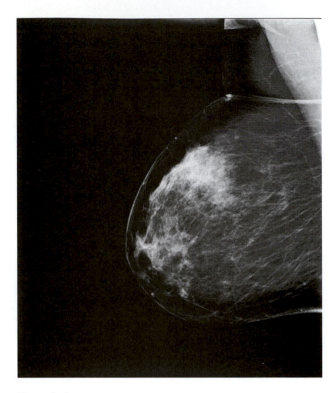

Figure 6–1

9. The MLO projection seen in Figure 6–1
   A. demonstrates sufficient pectoralis muscle
   B. demonstrates the entire breast adequately
   C. fails to demonstrate sufficient pectoralis muscle
   D. represents a camel's nose

10. Retroglandular fat space is located
    A. anterior to the pectoralis muscle and posterior to the breast tissue
    B. posterior to the pectoralis muscle
    C. posterior to the superficial fascia
    D. anterior to the mammary stroma

11. Which of the following would poorly image the lateral breast?
    A. ML
    B. XCCL
    C. LM
    D. MLO

12. Connective tissue that encapsulates the mammary stroma is referred to as
    A. retromammary fat
    B. fascia
    C. adipose tissue
    D. connective tissue

13. Full field digital mammography (FFDM) features which of the following functions as post-processing capabilities?
    A. Window leveling
    B. Film annotation
    C. Magnification
    D. All of the above

14. Following a ductogram, which of the following should be done prior to patient dismissal to prevent duct obstruction?
    A. Apply pressure to the breast to remove the contrast media
    B. Apply a wet dressing to the breast to absorb draining contrast
    C. Apply a dry dressing to the breast to absorb draining contrast
    D. Nothing needs to be done

15. Which type of cells line the terminal ductal lobular unit?
    A. Dermal cells
    B. Epithelial cells
    C. Acini cells
    D. None of the above

16. Small sac-like structures located within the TDLU responsible for milk production are referred to as
    A. epithelial cells
    B. intralobular ductal units
    C. acini
    D. TDLU

17. A malignancy that involves the epithelial cells of the TDLU but contains itself within the TDLU network describes
    A. adenocarcinoma
    B. invasive malignancy
    C. in situ malignancy
    D. microcalcifications

18. The plotted mid-density and the density difference values must fall within _____ of the control value.
    A. +/− 0.05
    B. +/− 0.10
    C. +/− 0.03
    D. +/− 0.40

19. The ACR requires a minimum of _____speck groups to be identified on the phantom image for analog imaging facilities.
    A. 2
    B. 3
    C. 4
    D. 5

20. Which of the following would not affect breast tissue density?
    A. Age
    B. Microcalcifications
    C. Hormone status
    D. Cyclic changes of menstruation

21. When a facility has received accreditation, the MQSA certificate is valid for
    A. 1 year
    B. 2 years
    C. 3 years
    D. 5 years

22. Mastalgia describes
    A. inflammation of the breast
    B. engorgement of the breast
    C. pain in the breast
    D. enlargement of the breast

23. Microcysts that contain a mixture of radiopaque particles mixed with fluid are referred to as
    A. popcorn type calcifications
    B. Milk of Calcium
    C. rim calcifications
    D. microcalcifications

24. Which of the following are characteristics of a potential malignant mass?
    1. A single microcalcification
    2. A cluster of microcalcifications
    3. A larger than 2 mm calcification
    4. Pleomorphic appearance
    A. 1 and 3
    B. 2 and 3
    C. 2 and 4
    D. 1 and 4

25. An overgrowth of epithelial cells in a way that is not normal is
    A. epithelial hypoplasia
    B. epithelial hyperplasia
    C. epithelial migration
    D. epithelial aplasia

26. A patient who presents with a warm, swollen breast with swollen lymph nodes and nipple inversion would be suspected of having
    A. LCIS
    B. DCIS
    C. Paget's disease
    D. (IBC) inflammatory breast cancer

27. Cancer occurrence in men is approximately
    A. 1%
    B. 5%
    C. 7%
    D. 9%

28. Patient motion on a film would be categorized as
    A. a processing artifact
    B. a film handling artifact
    C. an exposure artifact
    D. a static artifact

29. A large air-gap technique is applied in magnification imaging to
    A. reduce scatter and reduce contrast
    B. increase scatter and reduce contrast
    C. reduce scatter and improve contrast
    D. increase scatter and improve resolution

30. Tumors that are estrogen receptor negative
    1. will respond to tamoxifen treatment
    2. will not respond to tamoxifen treatment
    3. respond to the effects of estrogen
    4. do not respond to the effects of estrogen
    A. 1 and 3
    B. 2 and 3
    C. 1 and 4
    D. 2 and 4

31. The most common solid and benign mass within the breast is
    A. a cyst
    B. a papilloma
    C. an adenocarcinoma
    D. a fibroadenoma

32. The goal(s) of compression is to
    A. reduce OID of a lesion
    B. reduce radiation dose to the breast
    C. allow more uniform exposure of the breast
    D. all of the above

33. At what stage of cancer would a patient be with any T or N assignments along with M1?

    A. Stage 1

    B. Stage 2

    C. Stage 3

    D. Stage 4

34. Unilateral nipple discharge

    1. may indicate benign circumstances

    2. may indicate malignant circumstances

    3. can vary in color

    A. 1 and 2

    B. 1 and 3

    C. 2 and 3

    D. all of the above

35. Which of the following would increase the likelihood of radiographic mottle?

    A. Decreased screen speeds and high mAs

    B. Increased screen speeds and high mAs

    C. Increased screen speeds and low mAs

    D. Increased screen speeds and low mA

36. The dilated segment of a duct just before its emergence at the surface is referred to as

    A. duct ectasia

    B. ampulla

    C. nipple

    D. Morgagni's tubercles

37. When performing the darkroom fog test, the optical density difference between the adjacent fogged and unfogged areas of the film should not exceed _____.

    A. 2.20

    B. 0.10

    C. 0.05

    D. 0.005

38. Selection of kVp values may depend on

    A. radiologist preference

    B. calibration of equipment

    C. film-screen characteristics

    D. all of the above

39. Which of the following must be done in order to acquire CC ID view on a patient?

    1. Displace the implant anteriorly

    2. Displace the implant posteriorly

    3. Pull forward the surrounding breast tissue from the implant

    4. Apply compression to include partial implant

    A. 1 and 3

    B. 2 and 3

    C. 2, 3, and 4

    D. 1, 3, and 4

40. A halo sign is typically associated with

    A. microcalcifications

    B. a malignant lesion

    C. a benign mass

    D. atherosclerosis

41. Nipple inversion

    1. may be normal

    2. may be an indicator of underlying disease

    3. is always benign

    A. 1 and 2

    B. 2 and 3

    C. 1 and 3

    D. all of the above

42. If after examining a phantom image the density and the density difference readings exceed limits, which of the following should be investigated?

    A. The film batch

    B. The processor

    C. The unit's generator

    D. All of the above

43. The upper half of the right breast can be evaluated with BSE when the patient is

    A. upright

    B. supine

    C. RPO

    D. LPO

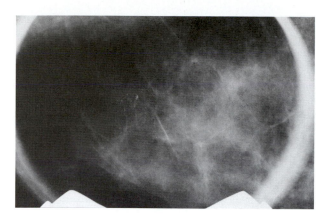

Figure 6–2

44. The pathology demonstrated in this coned magnification view, Figure 6–2, demonstrates
    A. papilloma
    B. duct ectasia
    C. microcalcifications
    D. cyst

45. The accuracy of mammography is approximately
    A. 50%
    B. 75%
    C. 90%
    D. 100%

46. What type of pressure should be administered with the pads of fingers 2, 3, and 4 during BSE?
    1. light
    2. medium
    3. deep
    A. 1 and 2
    B. 1 and 3
    C. 2 and 3
    D. All of the above

47. Inadequate breast compression may result in
    A. patient motion
    B. nonuniform exposure
    C. superimposition of structures
    D. all of the above

48. Hormonal treatment such as tamoxifen could be an option for patients who have a breast tumor which is
    A. estrogen receptor positive
    B. estrogen receptor negative
    C. progesterone receptor positive
    D. progesterone receptor negative

49. If the AEC detector is placed under a region of the breast that is composed more of adipose tissue than glandular tissue, the resultant image would demonstrate the glandular tissue
    A. as underexposed
    B. as overexposed
    C. with good exposure
    D. overpenetrated

50. Women over 50 should undergo mammography
    A. yearly
    B. bi-annually
    C. every other year
    D. every three years

51. Which quadrant of the breast has the highest incidence of breast cancer?
    A. UOQ
    B. UIQ
    C. LOQ
    D. LIQ

52. Which of the following describes a normal axillary lymph node?
    1. A fixed node about 3 cm
    2. Oval in shape
    3. Lucent center
    A. 1 and 2
    B. 1 and 3
    C. 2 and 3
    D. All of the above

53. Prognosis and/or treatment of a patient diagnosed with a breast lesion is determined by
    A. nodal involvement
    B. tumor size
    C. metastasis
    D. all of the above

54. The accumulation of clear fluid following a surgical procedure is
    A. hemangioma
    B. hematoma
    C. seroma
    D. galactocele

55. Which of the following could be a post-operative outcome of a mastectomy?
    1. Incisional pain
    2. Numbness of the underarm or chest wall
    3. Hematoma
    A. 1 and 2
    B. 2 and 3
    C. 1 and 3
    D. All of the above

56. Which of the following factors is the most predictive of breast cancer development?
    A. A multiparous mother
    B. A mother who has never breast fed
    C. Late menopause
    D. Age

57. According to the ACR/ACS guidelines, a baseline mammogram should be established
    A. at age 30
    B. at age 40
    C. at age 42
    D. at age 45

58. Which of the following projections are required for routine screening mammography?
    1. MLO
    2. CC
    3. True lateral
    A. 1 and 2
    B. 1 and 3
    C. 2 and 3
    D. All of the above

59. When correctly trying to position a CC projection, the patient's head should be
    A. straight ahead
    B. turned towards the breast being imaged
    C. turned away from the breast being imaged
    D. looking down

60. If positioning a standard CC projection and the nipple will not present in profile, how should the mammographer proceed?
    A. Do nothing; the radiologist will likely figure it out
    B. Take the film and leave a written notation for the radiologist
    C. Note it on the patient's history form
    D. Mark the nipple with a BB and attempt to reposition

61. In which of the following instances would the application of AEC not be recommended?
    A. MLO with implant displaced
    B. Large fibroglandular breasts
    C. CC with implant
    D. Post-biopsy patient

62. The most accurate modality to interrogate the integrity of an implant is
    A. mammography
    B. ultrasound
    C. nuclear medicine
    D. MRI

63. Breast reconstruction options include
    1. flap surgery
    2. implants
    3. TRAM flap
    A. 1 and 2
    B. 1 and 3
    C. 2 and 3
    D. All of the above

64. The MLO in Figure 6–3 demonstrates
    A. mammographically benign calcifications
    B. mammographically malignant calcifications
    C. speculated mass
    D. fibroadenoma

65. The breast tissue type seen in Figure 6–4 is
    A. dense glandular
    B. fibrofatty
    C. fibroglandular
    D. fatty

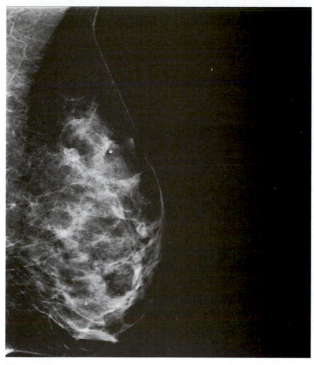

Figure 6–3

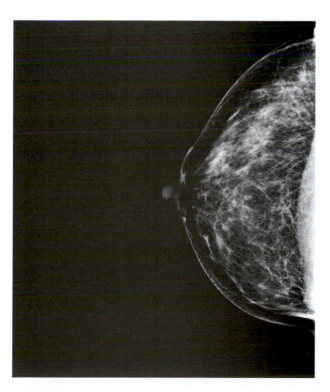

Figure 6–4

66. A patient with a prominent pacemaker could be accommodated with which of the following projections?
    A. CC and MLO
    B. CC and LMO
    C. CC and ML
    D. CC and AT

67. The "BB" on a TAN projection should be aligned
    A. parallel to the beam
    B. perpendicular to the beam
    C. superior to the beam
    D. obliqued to the beam

68. At what angle should the relationship be between the chest wall and the IMF when determining image receptor height for a CC position?
    A. 30 degrees
    B. 45 degrees
    C. 60 degrees
    D. 90 degrees

69. Artifacts could be categorized into
    A. screen related
    B. processing related
    C. equipment related
    D. all of the above

70. In which portion of the breast is a lesion located if it appears lower on a true lateral position compared to the MLO position?
    A. Anterior
    B. Inferior
    C. Lateral
    D. Medial

71. Which position could be utilized to assist in a tangential projection of a lesion in the medial breast region?
    A. LM
    B. AT
    C. CC
    D. MLO

72. Which of the following could be done to ensure maximum medial breast tissue on a large breasted patient is included on a CC projection?
    A. Have the patient hold onto both handles
    B. Have the patient turn her head away from the side being imaged
    C. Externally rotate the arm
    D. Pull opposite breast up and onto the bucky edge

73. A preoperative needle localization

    A. relies on excised specimen radiography

    B. marks the location of tissue to be examined

    C. is utilized in the instances of nonpalpable lesions

    D. all of the above

74. A patient who presents with unilateral spontaneous nipple discharge may undergo _____ to better assess the patient's condition.

    A. ductography

    B. pneumocystography

    C. FNA

    D. ultrasound

75. Which of the following would be a noninvasive means of evaluating axillary node involvement?

    A. Ultrasound

    B. Diagnostic views

    C. Scintimammography

    D. CAD

76. Blood supply to the breast is from the

    1. intercostal artery

    2. internal mammary artery

    3. lateral thoracic artery

    A. 1 and 2

    B. 2 only

    C. 2 and 3

    D. all of the above

77. To accurately acquire localization with spot compression views, the mammographer should

    A. measure posteriorly to the nipple to the level of the lesion

    B. measure anteriorly to the nipple to the level of the lesion

    C. measure posteriorly to the nipple to the level of the lesion and then attain a second measurement to the point of the lesion

    D. measure posteriorly to the nipple to the level of the lesion, then attain a measurement to the point of the lesion, then attain a third measurement from the lesion to the skin

78. The inferior medial breast may be better examined with which of the following projections?

    A. ML

    B. MLO

    C. LMO

    D. SIO

79. The IMF should absolutely be included on which of the following films?

    1. LM

    2. AT

    3. MLO

    A. 1 and 2

    B. 2 and 3

    C. 1 and 3

    D. All of the above

80. Computer aided detection is designed to:

    A. replace the need for a radiologist read

    B. be a wet read

    C. improve the accuracy of interpretation

    D. decrease productivity

81. On a MLO projection, the pectoralis muscle should appear

    A. thin and vertical

    B. convex to end at the level of the nipple

    C. concave to end at the level of the nipple

    D. rectangular

82. Which of the following quality control tests is evaluated monthly?

    A. Darkroom fog

    B. Visual checklist

    C. Phantom images

    D. Fixer retention

83. Which of the following is the required labeling for mammograms?

    A. A permanent patient ID

    B. Mammography unit indicator

    C. Cassette identifier

    D. All of the above

84. Which of the following would be a strong familial link(s) to breast cancer?

    1. mother

    2. sister

    3. paternal aunt

    A. 1 only

    B. 1 and 2

    C. 2 and 3

    D. all of the above

85. Which mechanism terminates the exposure when a predetermined amount of radiation is reached?

   A. kVp

   B. mAs

   C. AEC

   D. Density setting

86. The base plus fog value figured for daily processor QC should fall within

   A. +/− 0.10 of the established levels

   B. +/− 0.30 of the established levels

   C. +/− 0.003 of the established levels

   D. +/− 0.03 of the established levels

87. The comparative CC views seen in Figure 6–5 demonstrate which of the following breast tissue classifications?

   A. Glandular

   B. Fibroglandular

   C. Fibro-fatty

   D. Adipose

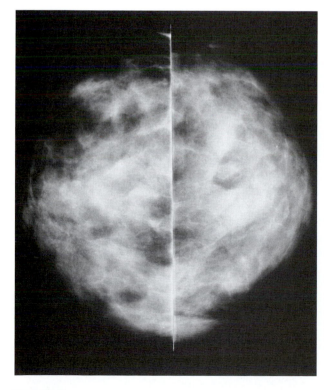

Figure 6–5

88. Before processing the sensitometric strip, the mammographer should

   A. check the developer temperature

   B. check the fixer temperature

   C. clean the viewboxes

   D. refill the processor with fresh chemicals

89. The background OD for phantom image should never vary by more than

   A. +/− 0.02

   B. +/− 0.20

   C. 1.02

   D. 1.40

90. A 36-year-old patient undergoing a reduction mammoplasty surgery should have a mammogram

   A. prior to the surgery

   B. following the surgery

   C. not until the age 40

   D. not until the age 45

91. Towels are advised for the compression test to

   A. protect the compression paddle

   B. protect the scale

   C. increase the amount of compression force applied

   D. simulate a compressed breast

92. To help compensate for reduced resolution during magnification imaging, which of the following should be implemented?

   A. Application of a small focal spot

   B. Application of a large focal spot

   C. Increase kVp

   D. Decrease mAs

93. The majority of breast cancers are located

   A. in the upper half of the breast

   B. in the lower half of the breast

   C. behind the nipple

   D. in the axilla

94. Daily processor QC will

   1. figure film contrast

   2. ensure quality film archival

   3. figure film speed

   A. 1 and 2

   B. 2 and 3

   C. 1 and 3

   D. all of the above

95. Technical factors set for phantom imaging should represent similar factors chosen to expose a _____ thick breast of 50:50 tissue distribution.

    A. 3.0–3.5 cm

    B. 2.0–2.5 cm

    C. 4.0–4.5 cm

    D. 5.0–5.5 cm

96. What target/filtration combination best penetrates a patient with dense breasts?

    A. Molybdenum target with molybdenum filtration

    B. Tungsten target with tungsten filtration

    C. Molybdenum target with K edge filtration

    D. Rhodium target with rhodium filtration

97. The anatomic structure identified as "A" in Figure 6–6 is

    A. pectoralis muscle

    B. subcutaneous fat

    C. retroglandular fat space

    D. deep fasica

98. An incident of AEC failure in which the film results in underexposure is due to

    A. processing overreplenishment

    B. excessive breast compression

    C. decreased film screen contact

    D. improper alignment of the AEC detector to the breast tissue

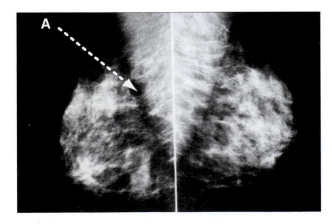

Figure 6–6

99. In DR mammography, the film and the cassette are replaced by:

    A. an intensifying screen

    B. a phospor plate

    C. a detector

    D. a laser

100. Which of the following patients is most likely to fall in the fibro-fatty breast tissue type category?

    A. Lactating mothers

    B. A 26-year-old male

    C. A young woman with 3 or more children

    D. A young woman age 28 with no children

101. The beryllium exit port window is necessary because

    A. the target produces high energy photons

    B. regular glass hardens the emerging beam

    C. regular glass softens the emerging beam

    D. of photoelectric interactions

102. Contrast of a breast image could be improved by

    A. reducing breast thickness

    B. application of grid imaging

    C. ideal processing conditions

    D. all of the above

103. Contrast and spatial resolution is improved with application of

    A. grids

    B. magnification views

    C. AEC

    D. compression

104. Reciprocity law failure may be seen with which of the following?

    A. Times longer than 1 second

    B. Times shorter than 1 second

    C. Times longer than 0.5 seconds

    D. Times shorter than 0.5 seconds

105. The rare tumor demonstrated in Figure 6–7 is likely a _____ based on its mammographic appearance.

    A. lipoma

    B. papilloma

    C. cystosarcoma phylloid

    D. fat necrosis

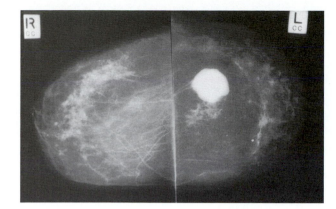

Figure 6–7

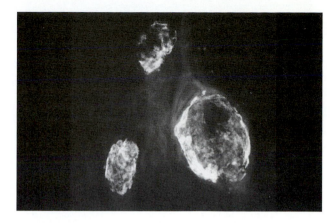

Figure 6–8

106. Which of the following characteristics would describe a likely benign mass?
1. Fatty composition
2. Solid composition
3. Circumscribed borders

A. 1 and 2

B. 1 and 3

C. 2 and 3

D. All of the above

107. Radiation therapy, chemotherapy, and/or tamoxifen would be considered

A. diagnostic tools

B. prevention agents

C. adjuvant therapy

D. cures

108. Collimating close to breast tissue margins is typically not applied to routine breast imaging as it will affect

A. radiopaque markings

B. image resolution

C. the contrast of an image

D. image viewing

109. The correct amount of molybdenum filtration added to a molybdenum target is

A. 0.03 mm

B. 0.3 mm

C. 3 mm

D. 30 mm

110. As the magnification factor increases, the _____ increases, and _____ decreases.

A. patient dose and resolution

B. patient dose and scatter

C. scatter and density

D. scatter and focal spot size

111. The pathology demonstrated in Figure 6–8 that may be a result of breast trauma or injury may be identified as

A. lipoma

B. hematoma

C. abscess

D. fat necrosis

112. The post-menopausal breast could be described as
1. varied densities
2. continued degeneration of fibroglandular tissue
3. increased adipose tissue

A. 1 and 2

B. 2 and 3

C. 1 and 3

D. all of the above

113. AEC may be used in all of the following projections on an analog mammography unit except

A. CV

B. specimen imaging

C. CC

D. AT

114. The majority of glandular tissue is located

A. central and medial

B. central and lateral

C. superior and lateral

D. inferior and lateral

115. The greatest advantage of digital mammography over conventional mammography is

    A. patient dose is increased due to the higher resolution of the digital image

    B. a reduction in positioning errors

    C. the digital image can never be transferred into a hard copy

    D. digital technology allows for image manipulation

116. Adipose tissue appears mammographically as

    A. tissue with more density

    B. tissue with less density

    C. tissue with equal density

    D. none of the above

117. A round, radiolucent lesion surrounded by a calcified rim is likely

    A. fibroadenoma

    B. Milk of Calcium

    C. cyst

    D. oil cyst

118. A H&D curve for a digital imaging system would appear

    A. with a steep slope

    B. with a shallow slope

    C. with no slope

    D. with a linear response

119. The left RL position requires the superior portion of the breast to be rolled

    A. medially

    B. laterally

    C. superiorly

    D. inferiorly

120. A "suspicious" finding on a mammogram means

    A. findings have a probability of being benign

    B. findings have a definite probability of being malignant

    C. findings have a high probability of being malignant

    D. additional evaluation is necessary

ANSWERS AND RATIONALES

1. **(B)** When too much of the patient's shoulder and axilla fall into the image receptor, inadequate compression will be applied to the inferior portion of the breast.

2. **(B)** The compression amount applied in the automatic mode should be between 25 and 45 lbs. Manual compression amounts applied will depend on the patient's breast size and tolerance.

3. **(C)** The sentinel node is the first lymph node that receives drainage from the tumor. This node can predict the presence or absence of disease in the remaining nodes.

4. **(D)** Estrogen is the responsible hormone for ductal proliferation and progesterone is responsible for lobular proliferation and growth.

5. **(C)** Breast tissue begins to atrophy medially and posteriorly and then starts laterally. The last region to undergo atrophy is around the nipple.

6. **(C)** When areas of density are smaller than 1 cm, no matter how numerous, the cassette can return to clinical use.

7. **(B)** With increased kVp values, a lower contrast scale is produced as scatter production increases and differential absorption decreases.

8. **(B)** A true lateral position of the breast is useful when determining the movements of lesions, air-fluid levels, or to identify the relationship of structures within the breast to the nipple.

9. **(C)** This MLO image fails to meet the criteria on several different aspects. The projection inadequately demonstrates the inframammary fold, the pectoralis muscle fails to extend to the level of the nipple, and a skin fold shows within the region of the axilla. For these reasons, the projection should be rejected.

10. **(A)** The retroglandular fat space is located just anterior to the pectoralis muscle. It separates the mammary stroma from the pectoralis muscle.

11. **(C)** The LM projection would better visualize the medial breast tissue as it is situated closer to the image receptor than the lateral breast tissue. The MLO, XCCL, and ML would all be better projections to visualize the lateral breast.

12. **(B)** Fascial layers encapsulate the breast tissue or stroma. The most posterior layer is called deep fascia and the more superficial layer is called superficial fascia.

13. **(D)** FFDM allows post-processing to be applied to the image. FFDM allows post-processing functions such as: tissue equalization, window leveling, magnification, image invert, annotations, and measurement of structures. Tissue equalization compensates for variable breast densities. Magnification is through an electronic zoom which may reduce the need for additional images. Image invert is converting the image to appear like a photo negative. Window leveling manipulates the dynamic range to alter image contrast. Annotations and measurements can also be applied to a film.

14. **(B)** A wet dressing is applied to the breast to absorb draining contrast from the breast to avoid obstruction.

15. **(B)** Epithelial cells line the inner surface of the TDLU.

16. **(C)** Acini located within the TDLUs are the milk producing units of the breast.

17. **(C)** In situ malignancies confine themselves to the membranes of the TDLU, while invasive carcinoma invades through the membranes and into the surrounding breast tissue.

18. **(B)** The plotted mid-density and density values should fall within $+/- 0.10$ of the control value and not exceed $+/- 0.15$.

19. **(B)** A minimum of four fibers, three speck groups, and three masses must be identifiable.

20. **(B)** Hormone status, age, number of pregnancies, cyclic monthly changes, and the involution process all alter the density of the breast tissue. Microcalcifications may present themselves within the breast with increased density, but overall will not affect the overall density of the breast tissue.

21. **(C)** The MQSA certificate is valid for a period of 3 years.

22. **(C)** Mastalgia is pain within the breast that may be cyclic or noncyclic. Pain in the breast is an unusual presentation. An underlying carcinoma doesn't usually present with pain until it is advanced.

23. **(B)** Milk of Calcium are microcysts containing a fluid-debris level and are considered to be a benign appearing calcification. Milk of Calcium calcifications can be distinguished by CC and ML projections. Rim calcifications occur along the borders of a benign mass. Popcorn type calcifications are large, dense, and irregularly shaped.

24. **(C)** Microcalcifications that are numerous, clustered, small, and pleomorphic (irregular in size and shape) are all suspicious characteristics.

25. **(B)** Epithelial hyperplasia is the initial increase in number of epithelial cells which can ignite a malignant disease process.

26. **(D)** Patients with IBC present with warm, swollen breasts, enlarged lymph nodes, pain or itching in the breast, and possibly nipple inversion. Due to the presenting symptoms of the patient, this is often misdiagnosed as mastitis. The patient may be treated as though it is mastitis, but will not respond to antibiotic treatment.

27. **(A)** Cancer in men is a very rare occurrence and occurs in approximately 1% of men.

28. **(C)** Patient motion would fall into the category of exposure artifact. Processing artifacts are specific to processor chemicals, roller quality, and workings of the mechanical elements. Film handling artifacts are specific to static and fingerprints.

29. **(C)** The large OID produced for magnification imaging will reduce the amount of scatter reaching the film and improve overall image contrast.

30. **(D)** Breast tumors are determined to be estrogen or progesterone receptors. Those tumors that test positive for estrogen receptors are more likely to respond to the effects of tamoxifen, as estrogen effects on the breast are now inhibited. Tumors that test negative for estrogen receptors will not respond to tamoxifen treatment and another treatment must be sought.

31. **(D)** Fibroadenomas are the most common solid, benign mass of the breast. They appear solid, uniform, and have clearly defined margins.

32. **(D)** Compression provides reduced thickness of the breast, therefore improving uniformity of exposure. Uniformity of exposure means that the OD differences correspond to the subtle attenuation differences in the breast, not to the differences in thicknesses of the breast tissue. Compression also allows OID of structures within the breast to be reduced, reduces patient motion and patient exposure.

33. **(D)** Stage 4 cancer is represented by any T (tumor) assignment, any N (node) assignment, and presence of metastasis (M).

34. **(D)** Unilateral discharge may indicate benign or malignant circumstances for the patient. Bilateral discharge is typically always benign and hormone related. Unilateral discharge that is either watery or bloody is associated more with carcinoma.

35. **(C)** When insufficient photons reach the film, especially with more sensitive films (increased speeds), the artifact radiographic mottle results.

36. **(B)** The dilation of the lactiferous duct before it emerges at the nipple is a point of reservoir referred to as the ampulla.

37. **(C)** The OD between two adjacent areas on the film should not exceed 0.05. Values greater than this indicate a potential problem that requires corrective action before processing further mammograms.

38. **(D)** Mammography units have the ability to increase or decrease kVp in increments of 1 kVp. Kilovoltage selection may be determined by a variety of factors such as: target/filtration materials, radiologist preference, the patient, equipment calibration, and film-screen characteristics.

39. **(B)** Proper positioning for the ID views requires the implant to be displaced posteriorly and the surrounding breast tissue to be pulled forward. Compression should be supplied to the actual breast tissue separated from the implant, but should not include the implant.

40. **(C)** A halo sign appears as a thin, curvilinear structure caused by compression of a mass upon surrounding fatty tissue. Generally, this is associated with benign lesions.

41. **(A)** Nipple inversion may be a part of normal development for a patient or it may be a relatively recent onset. Patients should be questioned of this and answers properly documented. Recent nipple inversion can be associated with an underlying carcinoma.

42. **(D)** If density and density difference readings exceed limits, then the processor, film batch, and the unit's generator should all be evaluated and corrected if necessary. A medical physicist should be contacted any time grid lines and/or grid artifacts continually occur. In addition, if an increased number of simulated test objects appear within the phantom the medical physicist should also be contacted.

43. **(A)** BSE should be performed in both upright and supine positions. Upright examination allows for evaluation of the upper half of the breast, while supine for the lower half of the breast. It is important to examine in both positions.

44. **(C)** Microcalcifications and their characteristics are better demonstrated through the application of coned magnification views. Microcalcifications less than 0.5 mm in size have a higher probability of

malignancy. Macrocalcifications are associated with benign processes and measure 2.0 mm or larger.

45. (C) Film screen mammography is not 100% accurate. It is approximately 90–93% accurate, as 7% of breast cancers are found through BSE or CBE.

46. (D) BSE should include three different pressure types to be delivered by the pads of the fingers. A light pressure to allow for palpation of more superficial structures, a medium pressure, and a deep pressure to allow palpation to the mid-breast and closer to the chest wall.

47. (D) Adequate compression is necessary as it reduces tissue thickness, separates structures within the breast bringing them closer to the film, provides a more uniform thickness of tissue for production of uniform density, reduces patient motion, reduces patient dose, and improves resolution.

48. (A) Tumor receptors reacting positively to estrogen would likely respond to a drug such as tamoxifen. Tamoxifen functions to block the estrogen receptors in the breast.

49. (A) As glandular tissue is of increased density, it will appear underexposed on the image when the adipose tissue is positioned over the AEC detector.

50. (A) Women 40 and over should undergo screening mammography yearly.

51. (A) The highest incidence falls in the quadrant with the highest amount of breast tissue. In addition, the UOQ is also a later area of the breast to undergo the involution process. The retroareolar area is the last area in the breast to undergo involution.

52. (C) Normal axillary nodes are sometimes visible on mammograms. The typical normal node is oval in shape, contains a lucent center, and is about 2 cm or less. Nodes that are enlarged, fixed, and have solid centers may be indicators of malignant disease, but could certainly be benign as well.

53. (D) Nodal involvement (N), tumor size (T), and metastasis (M) are components of the cancer staging to help in treatment plans and/or prognosis.

54. (C) An accumulation of clear fluid is known as a seroma. An accumulation of blood is a hematoma.

55. (D) There are a variety of after effects that post-mastectomy patients may experience. These could range from incisional pain or tightness to

the area, wound infection, hematoma, drainage tube, numbness to the underarm or chest wall from nerve damage, or weakening or stiffness of the shoulder and arm.

56. (D) Gender followed by age, genetics, family history, or a previous breast cancer occurrence are all classified as major risk factors that may be predictors for a patient.

57. (B) A baseline mammogram is typically established by age 40, or earlier if family history suggests.

58. (A) Routine screening mammography requires a CC and MLO to be acquired of each breast.

59. (C) The patient's head should be turned to look away from the side being imaged to prevent superimposition of structures over the breast.

60. (D) When nipples are not in profile, breast tissue should not be compromised to make the nipple appear in profile. The mammographer would be able to mark the nipple with a BB or take an additional view with the nipple positioned in profile. If the nipple is marked and/or NIP (nipple in profile) projection is acquired, the radiologist will not suspect a subareolar mass.

61. (C) AEC is not recommended for application when imaging a CC with the implant in place, as the detector will sense the density of the implant, resulting in a long exposure time.

62. (D) MRI is the best suited modality to interrogate the integrity of an implant. It is possible that ultrasound is an option. Implant ruptures can sometimes be small and lead to a small leak, therefore mammography is the unlikely modality of choice.

63. (D) Implants, Flap, or TRAM flap surgeries are all possible options for reconstruction. The Flap surgery takes skin, fat, and muscle from the abdomen, buttocks, or back to construct a new breast. The TRAM flap removes muscle, fat, and skin from the abdominal area to form a new breast. Patients who undergo the TRAM flap procedure will be considered for one of two types, either the pedicle or free flap procedure.

64. (A) The image represents scattered calcifications, many appearing as microcysts or Milk of Calcium. Milk of Calcium represents a mixture of fluid and debris that will change appearance between a CC and MLO projection.

65. (C) The image demonstrates a 50/50 distribution of fibroglandular tissue.

66. (B) Pacemaker patients could be imaged with standard CC and MLO projections. Pacemaker patients could be better accommodated with a CC and LMO to avoid contact of the compression paddle edge along the pacemaker.

67. **(A)** The BB marker should be positioned into view perpendicular to the image receptor therefore aligning parallel with the beam. Parallel alignment of the BB with the beam will allow the beam to skim across the region of the lesion.

68. **(D)** Between the chest wall and the IMF a 90 degree relationship should exist to ensure proper image receptor height for the CC position.

69. **(D)** Artifacts could be isolated to processing related artifacts, screen related artifacts, and equipment related artifacts.

70. **(C)** Medial lesions move more superiorly and lateral lesions move more inferior on a true lateral projection when compared to a MLO projection.

71. **(C)** From the CC position, the lesion within the medial segment could be rolled to position for the tangential beam.

72. **(D)** Bringing the opposite breast up and over the edge will help the patient bring more medial tissue along the chest wall of the affected breast without interference.

73. **(D)** The preoperative needle localization procedure is utilized in instances in which the patient has a nonpalpable lesion or a suspicious area noted on a mammogram. Localization assists the surgeon with removing the smallest amount of breast tissue to attain a specimen. Specimen imaging is required to verify correct removal of tissue.

74. **(A)** Ductography or galactography is a procedure that allows visualization of the ductal system which may localize the area of concern. The duct is isolated and cannulated, allowing introduction of a small amount of contrast into the ductal tree to allow visualization with mammography.

75. **(C)** Scintimammography has advanced to be a complimentary procedure to routine mammography. It may be useful when mammograms are inconclusive or if trying to assess axillary nodal involvement.

76. **(D)** Arterial blood supply to the breast comes from the lateral thoracic artery, which is a branch of the axillary artery, the intercostal arteries, along with the internal mammary artery which runs along the sternum.

77. **(D)** Proper lesion triangulation eliminates the guess-work in lesion localization.

78. **(D)** The SIO projection requires C-arm angulation of 45 degrees, allowing visualization of the upper inner and lower outer quadrant. The beam is directed from a superior lateral approach towards the inferior and medial breast.

79. **(C)** The MLO and true laterals are to include the IMF to ensure all breast tissue has been included on the film. The AT is a projection focused specifically to the axillary tail or the Tail of Spence and therefore may not include the IMF.

80. **(C)** CAD is designed to improve accuracy and productivity of a radiologist, not to replace the interpretation of the radiologist.

81. **(B)** A properly positioned MLO should evidence the pectoralis muscle in a convex configuration to extend from the axilla down to the level of the nipple. A pectoralis muscle that appears thin and vertical, concave, or triangular up at the level of the axilla all indicate improper tube angulation according to the pectoralis muscle.

82. **(B)** Visual inspection of the entire mammography unit according to the checklist should be performed each month.

83. **(D)** Required labeling on a mammogram includes a permanent patient identifier, R/L position markers, mammography unit indicator, cassette number, and mammographer identifier.

84. **(B)** First degree relatives such as mother, sister, daughter pose as strong familial breast cancer links.

85. **(C)** AEC is a device which is set at a predetermined level and will shut off when that level of exposure has been reached.

86. **(D)** Base plus fog must remain within +/− 0.03 of the established limit otherwise immediate corrective action must be taken. Base plus fog values may alter due to processing conditions such as replenishment, temperature, and chemistry.

87. **(A)** The extremely dense breasts demonstrated in the comparative CC views show very little percentage of other tissue densities.

88. **(A)** Upon stabilization of developer temperature, the developer temperature should be checked first, before running a processor QC strip.

89. **(B)** The OD of the phantom film should not be less than +/− 1.20 with the control limits being +/− 0.20. Therefore, it is suggested that an OD of 1.40 is optimal so the overall value would not fall below 1.20 in cases in which a -0.20 instance results.

90. **(A)** Patients under 35 years of age undergoing reduction mammoplasty surgery should have a mammogram prior to surgery to ensure there are no areas of suspicion before undergoing surgery. A baseline mammogram will then be established or reestablished following the surgery for future exam comparison.

91. **(A)** Towels are placed above and below the scale to provide protection to the cassette holder and compression paddle during the compression testing procedure.

92. **(A)** Focal spot blur will occur when changes between the source and the object occur, such as with magnification imaging. To compensate for this, the smallest focal spot should be employed to reduce the focal spot blur, and reduced resolution. Remember that resolution/sharpness is always reduced with magnification imaging.

93. **(A)** 74% of breast cancers are located in the upper half of the breast, the UOQ and UIQ together. Approximately 50% of cancers arise in the UOQ alone.

94. **(D)** The sensitometric step closest to 1.20 becomes the medium density or the speed step. The density difference becomes the contrast in-dicator. Daily processor quality control also ensures the day-to-day operations are stable.

95. **(C)** A testing phantom should simulate a 4–4.5 cm compressed breast with medium tissue glandularity.

96. **(D)** Rhodium possesses a slightly higher atomic number which produces KeV that are 2–3 higher than the molybdenum targets, allowing for better penetration of denser breast tissue.

97. **(C)** The radiolucent band that runs just anterior to the pectoralis muscle represents the retroglan-dular fat space.

98. **(D)** An AEC detector that isn't adequately placed completely under breast tissue or that fails to correspond to the densest portion of the breast may result in a shortened exposure and shuts off too soon to acquire enough exposure for the remaining breast tissue.

99. **(C)** In DR mammography, cassettes are no longer necessary, as the part is positioned over a detector. The detector converts the signal and sends it through a fiberoptic cable for viewing.

100. **(C)** Fibro-fatty breast consists of 50/50 adipose and fibroglandular tissue. Women between 30 and 50 years of age along with young women with 3 or more children fall within this category as well.

101. **(B)** Standard glass would harden the emerging beam. Beryllium is utilized to allow characteristic radiation to emerge from the tube and interact with the breast tissue for optimum production of the photoelectric effect in the breast.

102. **(D)** Contrast of an image could be improved by reducing breast thickness with adequate compression, applying grids, ensuring proper processing conditions, and using appropriate target/filter combinations.

103. **(D)** By reducing tissue thickness with compression, contrast is improved and structures within the breast are brought closer to the film, improving resolution.

104. **(A)** Reciprocity law failure may be seen with longer exposure times, as the film will no longer record an image with increased exposure times.

105. **(C)** Cystosarcoma phylloids are rare fibroepithelial tumors. In most instances they are benign and the mass is excised, but on occasion they can be malignant.

106. **(B)** Probable benign masses appear with smooth or well circumscribed borders, fatty composition, or encapsulated. Furthermore mass characteristics must always be correlated with the clinical history of the patient to aid in proper diagnosis.

107. **(C)** Adjuvant therapy is selected according to the tumor characteristics and axillary node involvement per each patient situation.

108. **(D)** Collimation is not desired in routine mam-mography as the density produced on the film surrounding the breast creates a masking effect to aid in image viewing.

109. **(A)** Molybdenum filtration for a molybdenum target is 0.03 mm while a rhodium target requires 0.025 mm of rhodium filtration.

110. **(A)** Magnification imaging increases the skin dose to the patient and decreases resolution. Less scatter reaches the film due to the increased OID.

111. **(D)** Areas of fat necrosis in the breast may be a result of injury or trauma to the breast. It is a be-nign process which results in the death of fatty tissue that encapsulates itself and demonstrates areas of calcification.

112. **(D)** With increasing age the breast gradually loses denser tissue which is gradually replaced with adipose tissue.

113. **(B)** Cleavage views require both breasts to be positioned atop of the bucky with moderate compression in order to visualize deep medial

lesions. The position of the photocells will likely fall in between the breasts, therefore will not have adequate coverage to acquire an appropriate exposure. To overcome this, the breasts may be offset in order to attain tissue coverage over the AEC cell. Specimen imaging would not be successfully imaged with AEC application with analog mammography units.

114. **(B)** Most glandular tissue is located in the central to lateral regions of the breast, specifically the UOQ extending into the axilla.

115. **(D)** The greatest advantage of digital imaging is the ability to manipulate the image. Digital imaging does not necessarily increase dose to the patient and images may still be printed as a hard copy if necessary.

116. **(B)** Adipose areas within the breast allow X-ray to pass easily through the tissue creating a dense or black area on the film. Glandular tissue appears as dense or white areas on the film with a lower OD reading.

117. **(D)** Oil cysts are a result of a fat necrosis possibly from a previous injury to the breast. They appear radiolucent with a calcified rim that resembles an egg shell. Fibroadenomas are a solid mass.

118. **(D)** Digital imaging systems will produce an H&D curve with a linear response to the exposure, unlike conventional imaging systems that produce a toe, straight line, and shoulder portions to the curve. Digital imaging has a wider latitude and represents the variety of breast tissue differences well. Digital imaging plots the values of the intensities detected in a linear fashion, unlike traditional film screen imaging which represents only a certain range of densities for contrast and loses contrast due to overexposure (shoulder) and underexposure (toe).

119. **(B)** Rolled lateral (RL) or rolled medial (RM) are utilized when breast tissue superimposes a lesion or area of interest. RL projections roll the superior region of the breast laterally and the inferior region medially from a standard CC position. RM projections roll the superior breast region medially and the inferior region laterally from a standard CC position. Again the RL and RM views are helpful to move dense breast tissue from an area of a suspicious lesion or may be implemented to truly determine if there is a lesion in fact present. If a density is still noted after the roll, then the area seen on the mammogram is real.

120. **(B)** "Suspicious" findings have a definite probability of being malignant for the patient. "Highly suggestive of malignancy" findings have a high probability of being malignant.

Internet Resources and Bibliography

INTERNET RESOURCES

American Cancer Society

www.cancer.org

Breastcancer.org

http://www.breastcancer.org/

Centers for Disease Control

http://www.cdc.gov

Food and Drug Administration

http://www.fda.gov

National Breast Cancer Foundation

http://www.nationalbreastcancer.org/

National Cancer Institute

http://www.cancer.gov/

Surveillance Epidemiology and End Results (SEER)

http://seer.cancer.gov/

Susan G. Komen Breast Cancer Foundation

http://cms.komen.org/komen/index.htm

U.S. Department of Health and Human Services

http://www.womenshealth.gov/

BIBLIOGRAPHY

American College of Radiography. (1999). Mammography Quality Control Manual. Reston, VA.

Andolina, V., et al. (2001). *Mammographic imaging: A practical guide* (2nd ed.). Philadelphia, PA: Lippincott Williams and Wilkins.

Carlton, R. & Adler, A. (2006). *Principles of radiographic imaging: An art and a science* (4th ed.). Clifton Park, NY: Thomson Delmar Learning.

Cowling, C. (1998). *Delmar's radiographic positioning & procedures,* volume II: Advanced imaging procedures. Clifton Park, NY: Thomson Delmar Learning.

Ikeda, D. M. (2004). *Breast imaging: The requisites.* Philadelphia, PA: Elsevier-Mosby.

Kopans, D. B. (1998). *Breast Imaging* (2nd ed.). Philadelphia, PA: Lippincott Williams and Wilkins Publishing.

Peart, O. (2005). *Mammography and breast imaging: Just the facts.* New York: McGraw Hill publishing.

Index

Please note that page numbers followed by "f" indicates the figure

4.0 PROTECTION AND SECURITY

4.1 The End User shall use its best efforts and take all reasonable steps to safeguard its copy of the Licensed Content to ensure that no unauthorized reproduction, publication, disclosure, modification, or distribution of the Licensed Content, in whole or in part, is made. To the extent that the End User becomes aware of any such unauthorized use of the Licensed Content, the End User shall immediately notify Delmar. Notification of such violations may be made by sending an e-mail to delmarhelp@cengage.com.

5.0 MISUSE OF THE LICENSED PRODUCT

5.1 In the event that the End User uses the Licensed Content in violation of this Agreement, Delmar shall have the option of electing liquidated damages, which shall include all profits generated by the End User's use of the Licensed Content plus interest computed at the maximum rate permitted by law and all legal fees and other expenses incurred by Delmar in enforcing its rights, plus penalties.

6.0 FEDERAL GOVERNMENT CLIENTS

6.1 Except as expressly authorized by Delmar, Federal Government clients obtain only the rights specified in this Agreement and no other rights. The Government acknowledges that (i) all software and related documentation incorporated in the Licensed Content is existing commercial computer software within the meaning of FAR 27.405(b)(2); and (2) all other data delivered in whatever form, is limited rights data within the meaning of FAR 27.401. The restrictions in this section are acceptable as consistent with the Government's need for software and other data under this Agreement.

7.0 DISCLAIMER OF WARRANTIES AND LIABILITIES

7.1 Although Delmar believes the Licensed Content to be reliable, Delmar does not guarantee or warrant (i) any information or materials contained in or produced by the Licensed Content, (ii) the accuracy, completeness or reliability of the Licensed Content, or (iii) that the Licensed Content is free from errors or other material defects. THE LICENSED PRODUCT IS PROVIDED "AS IS," WITHOUT ANY WARRANTY OF ANY KIND AND DELMAR DISCLAIMS ANY AND ALL WARRANTIES, EXPRESSED OR IMPLIED, INCLUDING, WITHOUT LIMITATION, WARRANTIES OF MERCHANTABILITY OR FITNESS FOR A PARTICULAR PURPOSE. IN NO EVENT SHALL DELMAR BE LIABLE FOR: INDIRECT, SPECIAL, PUNITIVE OR CONSEQUENTIAL DAMAGES INCLUDING FOR LOST PROFITS, LOST DATA, OR OTHERWISE. IN NO EVENT SHALL DELMAR'S AGGREGATE LIABILITY HEREUNDER, WHETHER ARISING IN CONTRACT, TORT, STRICT LIABILITY OR OTHERWISE, EXCEED THE AMOUNT OF FEES PAID BY THE END USER HEREUNDER FOR THE LICENSE OF THE LICENSED CONTENT.

8.0 GENERAL

8.1 *Entire Agreement.* This Agreement shall constitute the entire Agreement between the Parties and supercedes all prior Agreements and understandings oral or written relating to the subject matter hereof.

8.2 *Enhancements/Modifications of Licensed Content.* From time to time, and in Delmar's sole discretion, Delmar may advise the End User of updates, upgrades, enhancements and/or improvements to the Licensed Content, and may permit the End User to access and use, subject to the terms and conditions of this Agreement, such modifications, upon payment of prices as may be established by Delmar.

8.3 *No Export.* The End User shall use the Licensed Content solely in the United States and shall not transfer or export, directly or indirectly, the Licensed Content outside the United States.

8.4 *Severability.* If any provision of this Agreement is invalid, illegal, or unenforceable under any applicable statute or rule of law, the provision shall be deemed omitted to the extent that it is invalid, illegal, or unenforceable. In such a case, the remainder of the Agreement shall be construed in a manner as to give greatest effect to the original intention of the parties hereto.

8.5 *Waiver.* The waiver of any right or failure of either party to exercise in any respect any right provided in this Agreement in any instance shall not be deemed to be a waiver of such right in the future or a waiver of any other right under this Agreement.

8.6 *Choice of Law/Venue.* This Agreement shall be interpreted, construed, and governed by and in accordance with the laws of the State of New York, applicable to contracts executed and to be wholly preformed therein, without regard to its principles governing conflicts of law. Each party agrees that any proceeding arising out of or relating to this Agreement or the breach or threatened breach of this Agreement may be commenced and prosecuted in a court in the State and County of New York. Each party consents and submits to the nonexclusive personal jurisdiction of any court in the State and County of New York in respect of any such proceeding.

8.7 *Acknowledgment.* By opening this package and/or by accessing the Licensed Content on this Web site, THE END USER ACKNOWLEDGES THAT IT HAS READ THIS AGREEMENT, UNDERSTANDS IT, AND AGREES TO BE BOUND BY ITS TERMS AND CONDITIONS. IF YOU DO NOT ACCEPT THESE TERMS AND CONDITIONS, YOU MUST NOT ACCESS THE LICENSED CONTENT AND RETURN THE LICENSED PRODUCT TO DELMAR (WITHIN 30 CALENDAR DAYS OF THE END USER'S PURCHASE) WITH PROOF OF PAYMENT ACCEPTABLE TO DELMAR, FOR A CREDIT OR A REFUND. Should the End User have any questions/comments regarding this Agreement, please contact Delmar at delmarhelp@cengage.com.